Every Breath
I Take

Every Breath I Take

. . . . . .

A GUIDE TO LIVING WITH COPD

RICK HODDER, M.D.
WITH SUSAN LIGHTSTONE

Foreword by Alan McFarlane,
Canadian Lung Association

in association with

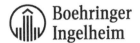
Boehringer
Ingelheim

Published in 2001 by Stoddart Publishing Co. Limited
895 Don Mills Road, 400-2 Park Centre, Toronto, Canada M3C 1W3

Distributed by:
General Distribution Services Ltd.
325 Humber College Blvd., Toronto, Ontario M9W 7C3
Tel. (416) 213-1919   Fax (416) 213-1917
Email cservice@genpub.com

05   04   03   02   01   1   2   3   4   5

Canadian Cataloguing in Publication Data

Hodder, Rick
Every breath I take: a guide to living with COPD

Includes index.
ISBN 0-7737-6144-6

1. Lungs — Diseases, Obstructive — Popular works. I. Lightstone, Susan. II. Title.

RC776.O3H63 2001   616.2'4   C00-932833-5

Cover design: Bill Douglas @ The Bang
Illustrations: Jeanne Simpson / Photographs: Robin Chernick
Text design: Tannice Goddard

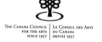

THE CANADA COUNCIL | LE CONSEIL DES ARTS
FOR THE ARTS | DU CANADA
SINCE 1957 | DEPUIS 1957

*We acknowledge for their financial support of our
publishing program the Canada Council, the Ontario Arts
Council, and the Government of Canada through the
Book Publishing Industry Development Program (BPIDP).*

Printed and bound in Canada

*To Mary and Jack, my mom and dad, for making me
proud when they listened to my youthful rantings and
stopped smoking before it was too late.
It's good to still have you here.*

*To Margo, Matthew, Tanis, and Jordyn, for making
every day a joy to live and for never starting to smoke.
Your love of life is exhilarating.*

*To those with COPD whom I've been privileged to know.
Your courage is uplifting and the lessons you teach invaluable.*
— R. V. H.

To the memories of Janet Jones and Edgar Boileau.
— S. L.

Contents

Foreword

*C*hronic Obstructive Pulmonary Disease (COPD) is a major cause of death and disability in Canada, affecting more than 750,000 Canadians, and there are strong indications that hundreds of thousands more are afflicted but undiagnosed. It is one of the few causes of death whose incidence has not decreased over the decades — in fact, a four-fold increase has been seen since 1971 — and it is looking like COPD will be mainly a women's disease in the new millennium.

Statistics, however, do not tell the true story of COPD. COPD can be best characterized as a disease of loss — loss of contact with people and the outside world, loss of control and confidence, loss of identity and self-worth, and loss of hope.

Yet it also inspires a search for renewed and newfound meaning. And that is what *Every Breath I Take* is all about: helping people with the illness maintain or re-create satisfying, joyful, and substantive lives. This book heralds a new era in the optimal management of COPD, and should certainly be required reading for anyone interested in providing the best, in care *and* prevention.

Over the upcoming months and years, many exciting developments in

COPD management promise to take shape that will help sufferers, their families, and their health care providers. The Lung Association has been significantly involved in the care of people with lung disease for years. Now, by focusing on COPD, we are evolving into the first place that those diagnosed with this disease can turn. We hope to facilitate the union of knowledge and expertise in COPD. Our first step was founding the Canadian COPD Alliance, a national organization created in 1998 that will strive to provide leadership to all those with a stake in COPD. We are now implementing a national support plan that will encompass a comprehensive approach to the disease, including a call centre with access to qualified counselors, new educational materials, and personal management programs.

Until this plan becomes a reality, *Every Breath I Take* points to the many community resources we currently have available.

The Lung Association commends the efforts of Rick Hodder and Susan Lightstone in providing a rich and balanced approach to a largely unknown subject. *Every Breath I Take* will inspire and teach everyone affected by COPD — physicians, allied health professionals, patients, family members, and associations like ours — so that together we can forge a new future for COPD patients, one that is bright and positive.

Alan McFarlane, Canadian Lung Association
December 2000

Acknowledgements

I owe the inspiration for *Every Breath I Take* to all the people with COPD I've been privileged to know over the years. After the medical interview is over and the "doctoring" completed, there's always time for talk. Talk about life, family, trips planned, about feeling optimistic, about feeling alone and isolated, about feeling scared — anything goes. I've learned that everyone brings something different and unique to the task of coping with COPD.

My COPD friends have amazing stories to tell — their ability and courage in meeting the challenges of COPD continually astonish me. The idea of telling the story of COPD through their experiences grew naturally from listening to them recount the details of their lives. With their help and the efforts of Susan Lightstone, *Every Breath I Take* was born. To all of you who taught me about the real nature of COPD — the human side — thank you.

Especially warm thanks to Arthur, Audrey, Don, Edgar, Janet, Jean, Lorraine, Louise, Mychelle, Peg, and Raymond for their time and generosity in sharing their stories with us.

Many colleagues contributed to *Every Breath I Take*. I offer huge thanks to Luanne Calcutt, Kim Danovitch, Mary-Jo Lewis, Debbie Swihart, and Karen Kinney for their aid in facilitating the patient interviews so essential to this project. From the beginning, Steve Simonot and Nozhat Choudry of Boehringer Ingelheim Canada Inc. encouraged our efforts and served as valued resources. Cindy Shcherban and Alan McFarlane of the Ontario Lung Association and Ross Reid of the Canadian Lung Association offered many helpful insights along the way.

Many people spent time and energy discussing issues and ideas with Susan and me. Thanks to Gay Pratt of Ottawa's Access Therapy Centre, Dr. John I. Stewart, Bob Elford, Kitty Wilkins of Statistics Canada, Brenda Hannivan of Port Perry's VitalAire, and Miriam Sobel, managing editor of the *Canadian Journal of Respiratory Therapy*. To everyone at Ottawa's Rehabilitation Centre — thank you. We're particularly indebted to Dr. Douglas McKim, Colleen Kenney, Maria Watson, Dr. Peter Henderson, and Dr. Meridith Marks.

They say a picture is worth 1,000 words and we were privileged to work with two talented artists who have made *Every Breath I Take* speak volumes. Thank you to Robin Chernick for her stunning photographs and to Jeanne Simpson for her clear, elegant drawings.

Editors are the people who make our work look easy. The Stoddart editorial team of Don Bastian, Sue Sumeraj, and Shaun Oakey enriched the book with their accurate and insightful comments. Thanks also to Bill Kretzel and Barbara Sibbald for their careful attention to our work.

For many years — almost as long as we've been friends — Susan Lightstone and I talked about writing a book together. Thank you, Susan, for ensuring that our book is now more than simply a "good idea."

Finally, this project was demanding of time and commitment. It would have been impossible without the patience and support of Margo, my true love, and that of our children, Matthew, Tanis, and Jordyn, our hopes for the future. I know Susan's family — Lyon, Adrian, and Nicola — provided the same loving and supportive environment for her. Without knowing it, my parents, Jack and Mary, and my mother-in-law, Kay, also provided important help as windows on a generation to which most of my COPD friends belong. They too are wonderful examples of how the human spirit can adapt to and overcome challenges.

Rick Hodder, Ottawa

Introduction

*B*reathing — we all do it. It's necessary for life. For most of us, it's easy to do, even when we exercise. It's so natural, we don't even realize we're doing it.

But for people with lung disease it's a different story. Every breath they take can be a struggle they must think about constantly, especially those afflicted with a disease called COPD. Chronic obstructive pulmonary disease — that's what COPD means — is a grab-bag term for a collection of diseases, emphysema and chronic bronchitis among them. All are characterized by chronic airflow limitation, or a difficulty in moving air into and out of the lungs easily.

Whether you're suffering from COPD or caring for someone who is, you know that COPD is all about catching a breath. And simply put, each and every breath counts. Easy breathing — something most folks take for granted — is often an enormous and debilitating struggle for those with COPD.

Given this fundamental fact of life that COPD patients and their caregivers face every day, we've decided to make *Every Breath I Take* a little different from what you might expect. Yes, you will find in the pages that follow all the latest medical information about COPD — which drugs might prove useful, and how to keep yourself fit and well nourished, for example. But we also want to give expression to the experience of living day in, day out with COPD. So we asked eleven people who have COPD to share their stories with us — and with you.

The profiles of these individuals convey how each has learned to cope with the progression of their disease, chronicling the changes they've made to their lives, the choices they've faced, their successes and their failures. You'll also meet caregivers and partners. People with COPD do not live in isolation, and the disease can have a profound impact on family members who may find themselves cast in the role of caregiver.

As you read through *Every Breath I Take,* you'll discover these voices of experience integrated with the topic of each chapter, telling us about COPD through the eyes of people experiencing the disease. We hope their stories and the practical advice they provide will put a human face on COPD that is both encouraging and informative — like a portable support group in book form. Most important, we want you to know that you're not alone in facing the challenges that life with COPD presents. Like the name says, COPD is a chronic disease. Once you've got it, you can't get rid of it. When you're suffering from a chronic disease like COPD, both you and your family face an uncertain and difficult future.

Even though most healthy people have never heard of COPD, it causes significant suffering in North America and around the world. The World Health Organization has estimated that by 2020 COPD will be the third leading cause of death worldwide. It currently ranks fourth among the leading causes of death in Canada and, as of 1997, fourth among the leading causes of death in the United States. More than 100,000 Americans die each year from COPD, while nearly 16 million are afflicted with the disease. And more than 750,000 Canadians (3 percent of the adult population) suffer from COPD, at a cost of several billion dollars annually to the health care system. But the emotional and physical cost to the individual cannot be measured in dollars and cents.

COPD is a smoker's disease. It's not usually diagnosed until patients are in their fifties or sixties. The statistics bear this out: the prevalance of COPD among Canadians thirty-five to fifty-four years old is 1.9 percent, but it leaps to 6.4 percent in the sixty-five- to seventy-four-year-old age group. Despite a decrease in the number of people smoking cigarettes,

COPD prevalence and mortality rates are on the rise. COPD is having a big impact on women in Canada — probably because of increased smoking in this group — and it is projected that by 2005 more women than men will be dying from COPD.

Despite these grim statistics, there are plenty of people living with the disease and many of them are doing remarkably well. As a measure of the magnitude of the impact of COPD in Canada, in March 1999 The Lung Association helped create a national forum called the Canadian COPD Alliance to "facilitate the development and implementation of national strategies for the prevention, early detection, and optimal management of COPD in Canada" (www.lung.ca/CCA/).

COPD is a complicated and perplexing affliction — indeed, the emotional toll of the disease can be as debilitating as its physical symptoms. This frustrating state of affairs is compounded by the widely held perception that COPD is a "self-inflicted" disease. Perhaps this attitude is one of the reasons why medical research into COPD has lagged behind that devoted to other pulmonary conditions such as asthma, with the result that available drug treatments have not had much positive impact on the treatment of COPD. In fact, many doctors still regard and treat COPD as if it were just "tough asthma," offering up the same drugs for both diseases. Such attitudes are changing as we learn more about the disease, thanks to new research initiatives.

Today, however, smoking cessation still remains the only hopeful means of altering the progression of COPD. We don't need to tell you how difficult it can be to kick the habit, but we'll strongly urge you to do just that in our chapter on smoking cessation.

There are many ways to manage your disease and, in turn, control and relieve your symptoms. As you progress through *Every Breath I Take*, you'll learn that this concept of "managing" the disease is unique to each individual — as the testimonies of our group of eleven illustrate. Depending on your experiences with COPD, your personal strategy can involve choosing a doctor who's right for you; getting adequate exercise; learning to breathe properly; preparing yourself to travel the world; eating nutritiously; maintaining a healthy weight; keeping tabs on your lung function; finding a rehabilitation program tailored to your needs; managing the stress associated with a chronic illness; and maintaining a close and intimate relationship with loved ones.

But the process of effectively managing your COPD starts with education. You need to know the what, how, when, and why of various techniques that can keep your COPD under control.

Each and every member of our group of eleven told us that learning about their disease was the first — and most important — step in living with COPD. We feel Raymond expressed it best. At seventy-four, he maintains an active lifestyle despite a diagnosis of COPD several years ago. A large medical encyclopedia sits prominently on a bookcase in the living room of his tidy apartment. Raymond refers to it often, refreshing his memory of the details of how various parts of his body work — or, as the case may be, don't work. "If you want to live with COPD and enjoy your life, you have to accept the disease. Once you've accepted it, you can begin to learn to adapt to it," he explains. "A big part of adapting to the disease is learning about it. And that means learning about how your body works.

"When I was first diagnosed with COPD, I went through hell. I was panicky. I didn't want to leave my apartment. I was afraid. My dad had died of COPD. Once he was diagnosed, he never left the house. I knew I didn't want to live the rest of my life like that. When I started to learn how my body worked, I learned what my lungs could and couldn't do for me. In other words, I started to learn my limits. I learned how far I could go. I learned how to breathe properly and how to listen to my body. But first, I had to sit down and think about things. When you're well, who cares? Your body works and you don't have to give it a second thought. But when it doesn't work well, you better start learning!"

So, how can you put *Every Breath I Take* to best use in learning about your disease? If you've just been diagnosed with COPD, you'll probably want to read it cover to cover. But each chapter is designed to stand alone as well. If you've been living with COPD for years and you're interested in learning only about the benefits of oxygen therapy, for example, head for chapter 11. If you're thinking about travelling to South Carolina for the winter, start with chapter 12. If it's time to get into shape, look at chapters 7 and 8. And so on. Refer to the table of contents, and use the index to find the topics that interest you.

Education, it has been said, is the movement from darkness to light. We hope *Every Breath I Take* will shed the light you need on the subject of COPD.

1

Catching Your Breath —
How the Lungs Work

"You can't understand it unless you've experienced it." That's Peg talking about breathlessness caused by COPD. "You think you're not going to get your next breath. You think your lungs will shut down. You're certain you'll die — right then and there. When I first started experiencing breathlessness, I'd panic. I had to get help right away. I had to find *someone* to help me." So, with each attack of breathlessness, Peg would rush to the nearest emergency department, looking for that someone to help her.

That was Peg's pattern for a couple of years — out of control and driven by panic — until her doctor suggested she start learning about her condition. An understanding of how her lungs worked, he suggested, would help her break her pattern of panic.

Peg took her tentative first steps by attending a respiratory rehabilitation program. "The key thing I learned," she says, "was that *I* am the someone who can help me. An integral part of that lesson came from learning the basic mechanics of the lungs — how they work and why they work that way. I now know that breathlessness is a symptom of COPD. By itself, it's not going to kill me. So, instead of running to the hospital,

I've stabilized my condition and learned to cope with many things on my own. I realize now that many of my fears about my health were fears of the unknown. With knowledge, I've conquered those fears. In the beginning, I only reacted to feelings. Now, I understand *why* I feel the way I do."

Understanding your COPD is your first step toward controlling and stabilizing its progress. Like Peg, you too can conquer your fears of the unknown with knowledge. You may not have the option of attending a respiratory rehabilitation program, but you can acquire that knowledge from many other sources, including this book. So, let's begin at the beginning. An understanding of COPD begins with a tour through the normal lung.

Breathing and Life

The **respiratory system** — your airways and lungs — is a complicated, sophisticated, and very delicate system. Like any sophisticated machine, the respiratory system can easily be messed up — and sometimes impossible to repair. When it's working well, this machine functions effortlessly. Every day, the average healthy person takes more than 17,000 breaths, automatically and easily.

Without the oxygen you take in with every breath of air, you would die within a few minutes. Your body needs energy to live, and every cell in your body requires oxygen to extract that energy from food molecules. Since your body cannot store oxygen for more than a few seconds, you have to keep breathing. It's a simple equation: no oxygen = no energy = no life. And your respiratory system is responsible for bringing in the air, about 20 percent of which is oxygen. But that's only half the process.

When oxygen combines with food molecules to release energy, two waste products are produced: carbon dioxide and water. Ridding carbon dioxide from the body is just as important as bringing in oxygen. If it isn't removed from your body, carbon dioxide will eventually poison you. So, just as oxygen must come in, carbon dioxide must get out, and to do so it travels up the same respiratory path that brings the oxygen in.

The respiratory system is all about the exchange of these two gases. Oxygen is inhaled into the body; carbon dioxide is exhaled. The exchange of these two gases takes place at the very end of the respiratory system, through a process called **diffusion**. From the point when you first breathe in an oxygen molecule to the final point where it diffuses into a cell is a long journey. Let's take that trip through the respiratory system.

Breathe in. You take air in through either your mouth or your nose. Both your mouth and nose do a pretty good job of filtering out large particles — dust and bacteria, for example — from the air you inhale. Those particles are trapped in the hairs in your nose and the mucus-producing membranes of your nasal passages and the large airways of the lungs. Those **mucous membranes** contain mucus-producing glands and are lined with **epithelial cells** that have short hairlike structures, called **cilia**, on their surfaces.

The cilia are constantly moving, sweeping along the mucus that contains many of the foreign particles you've breathed in. That sweeping motion carries the mucus away from your lungs. (Most of it ends up in your stomach because you swallow it.) Together, the cilia and mucus create an efficient filtration system, ensuring that the delicate lungs are not contaminated by dirty air. (As you'll learn later, one of the many harmful effects of cigarette smoke is to paralyze these cilia, causing inflammation that ultimately destroys them. When this happens, the mucus can't move along the airways; the mucus builds up until you are forced to cough it out. We call this **chronic bronchitis**.)

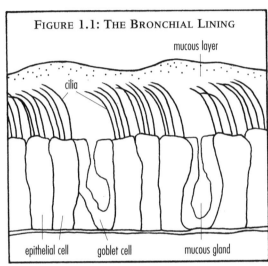

FIGURE 1.1: THE BRONCHIAL LINING

mucous layer

cilia

epithelial cell   goblet cell   mucous gland

The air moves along, entering your **pharynx**, the space at the back of your mouth, behind your nose. Food moves through your pharynx too, but is kept out of your lungs by a small trapdoor valve called the **epiglottis**. Below the pharynx, and protected by the epiglottis, is the **larynx**. The larynx is the upper portion of the main windpipe, or **trachea**. You can locate your larynx by feeling your neck for the bump that is your **Adam's apple**, a large band of gristle-like material called **cartilage** that protects the larynx from injury. (Your Adam's apple is named after the biblical Adam. While in the Garden of Eden, Adam is said to have got a piece of the forbidden fruit — the apple — stuck in his throat . . . hence the lump.) The larynx is also your voice box, containing your vocal cords. The nose, pharynx, and larynx make up the **upper respiratory tract.**

The **lower respiratory tract** starts just below the Adam's apple. The air continues to move down through the trachea, which is held open by rings of **cartilage.** Cartilage is a strong and resilient substance designed for double duty: it helps to protect the airways and keep them open. Grab your nose between your thumb and index finger, just where your nose joins your upper lip. Wiggle it from side to side. This structure separating your nostrils is also cartilage.

The trachea is about 12 cm long and about the same diameter as your thumb. At its end, it divides into two large airways called **bronchi** — the left and right main bronchi. Like the trachea, the bronchi are made up of muscular tubes lined with mucous membrane, a soft, pink tissue like the inside of your nose. The mucous membrane contains many mucus-producing glands as well as epithelial cells lined with cilia. These glands secrete the liquid mucus that keeps the airways moist. Like the trachea, the major bronchi are partly surrounded by cartilage.

The next stop for your breath of air is the lungs themselves. Visualize two sponges, each about the size of a football. That's what the lungs look like from the outside. Each lung is covered with a thin layer of tissue

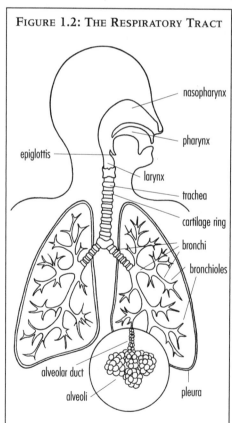

FIGURE 1.2: THE RESPIRATORY TRACT

nasopharynx
pharynx
epiglottis
larynx
trachea
cartilage ring
bronchi
bronchioles
alveolar duct
alveoli
pleura

called the **pleural membrane**. When this membrane is infected or inflamed, it causes pain — **pleurisy**. Each lung sits in an airtight cavity, the **pleural cavity** or chest cavity, like a sponge inside a sealed Mason jar. The lungs contain hundreds of thousands of tiny tunnel-like air passages. With all of its many branches, this network of branching tubes looks somewhat like an upside-down tree. In fact, the system of bronchi within the lung is called the **bronchial tree**. The lungs are divided into small sections called lobes. There are five lobes in all, three on the right and two on the left (to leave room for your heart). Each of these lobes is supplied by a major bronchus.

The two main bronchi keep on dividing into smaller and smaller **bronchioles**, forming the bronchial tree. The cartilage gradually thins out as the branching proceeds, and out in the periphery of the "lung-tree" the tiniest bronchioles are no longer supported by cartilage.

These tiny bronchioles, called the **terminal bronchioles**, are just 0.2 mm in diameter. That's about the size of the eye of a small sewing needle. The terminal bronchioles continue to branch, but at this stage they no longer resemble actual tubes; they are more like little bubbles of delicate tissue and look something like clusters of thin-walled grapes. These are the **alveolar ducts** and the **alveoli**. (The Latin word *alvus* means hollow belly.)

When we talk about one single alveolus, we're talking about a very tiny item. You'd need a microscope to see it. But there are a lot of them. A baby is born with about 20 million alveoli, and that grows to 300 million by the time the child is eight. This means that you have an enormous area in your lungs available for the diffusion of gases — more than 150 square metres. If all the alveoli in your body were spread out flat, they would cover an area about the size of a tennis court.

Many of the epithelial cells lining the bronchi and bronchioles have cilia. These cells perform just like their counterparts in the upper respiratory system, trapping foreign particles that make their way into the lung and moving them back up to the pharynx. The air must be as clean as possible to protect the delicate alveoli that are the final destination of the breath of inhaled air.

The real work of the lungs occurs in the alveoli. This is where diffusion — the transfer of oxygen and carbon dioxide — happens. Each alveolar duct opens out to about thirty alveoli. Each alveolus is surrounded by tiny blood vessels called **capillaries**. (To see what capillaries look like, look at the whites of your eyes in a mirror and see the blood vessels there.) The exchange of oxygen and carbon dioxide molecules occurs across the wall of each alveolus, which is only one cell thick. The oxygen molecules that have been breathed in **diffuse** into the blood circulating in the capillaries. Carbon dioxide, which has been generated in all the cells of the body during the energy-making process, diffuses from the blood into the alveoli. Then it's exhaled from the body, travelling out through the bronchioles to the bronchi and trachea and, finally, escaping via the nose and mouth. The newly oxygenated blood meanwhile travels away from the lungs to the heart, which pumps it around the body to supply the tissues.

Control of Breathing

What makes this system work? Breathe in. You thought about taking that breath, didn't you? That's unusual. You normally inhale and exhale with-

RAYMOND

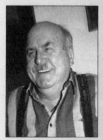

Raymond attends every workshop, lecture, or talk he can find on the subject of COPD. Several years ago his family doctor diagnosed him with COPD. But it wasn't until early 1999, when a serious lung infection forced him into hospital, that Raymond developed a respect for the power of his disease. "It was as if I'd been wandering around in a dark house," he explains. "I was tripping over things. If I only could turn on the light, I'd find my way." For him, the light was education. He now reads anything he can lay his hands on that concerns COPD. He takes careful notes. He heads down to the local Lung Association once a week to exercise and meet with a group of COPD patients. "This is my job now," he says. "I live alone. I need to learn all that I can to help myself stay healthy."

A look at Raymond — stocky and well fed — together with an examination of his refrigerator door — covered with recipes clipped from newspapers — reveals a man who loves his food. "Food has always been an issue for me," he admits. "Even more so now. My weight affects my breathing." The excess bulk he is carrying at his waist pushes up on his diaphragm, making the space designed to house his lungs smaller than it should be. This means Raymond's lungs can't expand as much as they need to when he inhales, resulting in breathlessness. Raymond also has non-insulin-dependent diabetes.

He's found that doctors aren't much help when it comes to the level of detail he likes to know. "It's all very well for the doctor to tell you to lose weight," Raymond says. "It's another thing to figure out how to do that. So I've spent my time learning about my diseases. It's the only way to look after yourself and, in my case, if I don't do it, nobody else will." Sure enough, there's a large, well-thumbed medical dictionary in his living room. "But I've had help too," he continues. He signs up for every local event he can find on diabetes and COPD. He's now enrolled in a course offered by the local Canadian

out thinking about it. The **respiratory centre** in your brain does that for you automatically. Think of the respiratory centre as information central. All the details of your respiratory system end up here. And that's a lot of information.

Here's an example. You're sound asleep and breathing normally. In other words, you're not thinking about breathing. While you're sawing logs, your respiratory centre is sending messages to your breathing muscles — the **diaphragm** and the **intercostal muscles** (the muscles of your chest wall that are located between your ribs). These muscles are **involuntary**. In other words, you don't have to think about making them work. An order from the respiratory centre telling those muscles to contract means that your chest cavity will expand, bringing air into your airways and down to the alveoli. When your respiratory centre orders the muscles to relax, your chest cavity shrinks, sending air out of your lungs.

Diabetes Association. He asks questions of the respiratory therapist who leads the S.O.B. (Shortness of Breath) Club he attends at the Ottawa branch of The Lung Association. He asks questions of the other COPD patients he sees at these meetings: What drugs are they on? What exercises work for them? How do they deal with breathlessness?

When his family doctor offered him a referral to the local pulmonary rehabilitation centre, Raymond jumped at the chance. In 1999, he spent two days a week for twelve weeks at the program, learning exercises, building up his strength and endurance, and — perhaps most important for Raymond — learning about nutrition.

Adult learning is nothing new for Raymond. After a career spent hiking through the bush of northern Canada locating ore bodies for mining companies, he came south in 1972 looking for a desk job. "I knew back then that I was having breathing problems. The cold was impeding my breathing, I was always coughing and short of breath. I was in my late forties and I knew if I waited too long I'd never be able to get another job. But to get a good job, I had to go back and finish high school." He did and ended his career working for the federal civil service, retiring in 1988. Along the way, he raised two children and divorced.

After his retirement, Raymond focused his energies on quitting smoking. "I'd smoked for over fifty years. I was so hooked. I'd tried to quit quite a few times but I couldn't make it work, even though my family doctor kept telling me that I *must* quit. Finally, I tried the patch. By that point, I'd made up my mind. I wanted to break the smoking pattern. But I needed the extra help of the nicotine the patch provided. It worked for me."

Now seventy-four, Raymond is philosophical about his health issues. "I never expected I'd live this long. The key thing I've learned from all this is that you have to accept what you've got to work with and you have to adapt to your new situation. A big part of adaptation is taking the responsibility to learn about yourself, your body, and your medical problems."

Your body is always monitoring the levels of carbon dioxide and oxygen in your blood. This task is performed by clumps of cells called **chemoreceptors** located at specific sites within your arteries. Your brain also tracks your blood pressure, how much effort your breathing muscles have to generate to make each breath, and how much air you've taken in with each breath. And all this is done without your having to give it a thought.

There are times when your conscious brain intervenes, however. Make yourself breathe in again. That's one example of a voluntary breath. Here's another. It's a hot day and you've walked too quickly. You begin to pant. At first you're not really aware that your breathing has become a bit heavier. Your panting is involuntary at this point. But then you start controlling your panting, trying to make it a bit more efficient. That's voluntary breathing.

It's natural to think about your breathing when you're exercising. But even then, your body will adjust your breathing on its own, without your intervention. When you exercise, your breathing speeds up. That's because you're burning oxygen to provide energy and producing more carbon dioxide that must be exhaled. Remember our equation, no oxygen = no energy = no life? The chemoreceptors alert the respiratory centre in the brain. The brain sends the message to your diaphragm and intercostal muscles to start contracting and relaxing faster. And you start breathing more quickly and bringing in more air with each breath.

On the opposite side of the coin, when you're sleeping, your energy needs are reduced. The respiratory centre slows the activities of the muscles. Your breathing becomes shallower and slower.

The Mechanics of Breathing

What exactly happens to your diaphragm and intercostal muscles when they get a message from the respiratory centre to inhale? To take a breath in, your chest needs to expand, filling the lungs with air. This happens in two ways — **diaphragmatic breathing** and **chest wall breathing**. The diaphragm is your main breathing muscle. You can't feel it, but it sits at the base of your chest, separating your lungs from your abdomen. It's shaped like a dome. When it contracts, the dome of the diaphragm moves downward, making the chest cavity expand, which pulls air into the lungs. The lungs stretch to accommodate the inhaled air. In much the same way, when certain intercostal muscles between the ribs contract, the ribs move up and away from the body. This action also expands the chest cavity and pulls air into the lungs.

When you exhale, everything relaxes and the process is reversed. Relaxing the muscular diaphragm allows the stretched lungs to relax, like a rubber band resuming its natural length after being stretched. The elastic lungs and chest wall contract, forcing air and carbon dioxide out of the body via the bronchi. Relaxing your chest muscles moves your ribs down and in. This, too, reduces the size of the chest cavity.

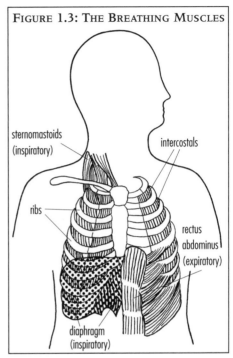

FIGURE 1.3: THE BREATHING MUSCLES

sternomastoids (inspiratory)

intercostals

ribs

rectus abdominus (expiratory)

diaphragm (inspiratory)

But there are other ways to force air out of your lungs. **Sneezing** and **coughing** are two examples. They also serve the useful purpose of helping to remove foreign particles from your lungs and nose.

Let's say you have a cold or bronchitis. As a result of your illness, you have too much mucus in your airways and it needs to be cleared. The single most effective way to clear the lungs is to cough. A cough is nothing more than an exaggerated big breath in followed by a forceful exhalation. But there's one interesting wrinkle. Following your big breath in, the larynx closes briefly while the exhalation begins. Since no air can move out through the closed larynx, pressure builds up in your lungs and airways. Then, at a critical point in time, the larynx opens. At precisely the same moment, the muscles of your abdominal wall (those "abs of steel") contract. These two actions serve to forcefully expel the air and mucus rapidly out of the airways and (ideally) into a tissue or handkerchief.

A cough is very forceful. Mucus coughed from the lungs has been clocked at 1,000 km/h! Excessive coughing can even break a rib if your bones are thin.

Coughing can be helpful if there is excess mucus to expel, but it can also be a real nuisance if the cough is **irritative**. An irritative cough is caused by excessive inflammation of the walls of your airways. An irritative cough often accompanies asthma or a viral cold, even though there may not be much mucus to expel. Inflammation irritates nerves in the airways that in turn send signals to the brain's cough centre, causing a cough or even paroxysms of coughing.

Sneezing is like an involuntary cough, but with a few interesting differences. The stimulus for a sneeze comes from an irritation of nerves in the nasal passageways, usually caused by inhaling some noxious particles (strong perfume or dust, for example). Once stimulated, the nasal nerves send a message to the cough centre of the brain and the entire cough sequence is initiated. Only this time, most of the expelled air is channelled up through the nose in an attempt to remove the offending particles. One of the more intriguing aspects of the sudden phenomenon of a sneeze is that the nerve impulses and violent reaction are similar to what happens during a sexual orgasm!

Measuring a Breath

When you're breathing normally, about five to seven litres of air move in and out of your lungs every minute. **Tidal volume** is the amount of air that enters your body when you take a normal, unforced breath in. Only about half of the air drawn in will make the entire journey down to the alveoli. Once you've breathed out in a normal, unforced way, you'll still have approximately three litres of air left in your lungs. This is your **resting respiratory level**, or **functional residual capacity**. But if you force things — for example, when you exercise — you can always inhale and exhale more than you normally do.

Here's an interesting fact. You can never completely empty your lungs of air. Even when you try to force all the air out of your lungs, some air always remains behind to keep your lungs partially inflated. This is called the **residual volume** and if you didn't have some residual volume left in your lungs, they would completely collapse. Another commonly used term is the **vital capacity** of your lungs. This is the maximum amount of air that you can exhale following a maximum inhalation. Measuring vital capacity is an important indicator of how well your lungs are functioning. (We'll talk about testing and diagnostic procedures in chapter 4.)

As we said at the beginning of this chapter, the respiratory system is sophisticated and complicated. That means the information you've just read is also fairly complicated. You might want to take Raymond's approach to learning about COPD. He has his medical encyclopedia within easy reach because he refers to it often. He reads and rereads to make sure he hasn't forgotten any details. As you learn more about COPD through the experiences of the members of our group, you might want to revisit this chapter for the basics of how the lungs work.

2

What Is COPD?

"*A*re you still smoking?"

Lorraine's family doctor greeted her with that question every time she had an appointment with him. "I'd even see him take a peek into my open purse, looking for cigarette packs," Lorraine recalls. "Every chance he'd get, he'd tell me it would be really good for me to quit. By then, I'd been smoking for at least twenty-five years. The things he said to me about quitting went in one ear and out the other. Finally, he told me: 'Lorraine, if you don't stop smoking now, you'll be sitting with an oxygen tank in five years.'" That was in 1989.

That final warning prompted Lorraine to quit smoking, but it was too late. She felt fine for the next five years. Then, in 1994, she experienced her first bout of debilitating breathlessness. That same year, her family doctor sent her to a respirologist, who diagnosed her COPD. She's been hooked up to an oxygen tank since September 1997. Today, she is waiting for a lung transplant. Her family doctor was off in his prediction by three short years.

Lorraine's long history of cigarette smoking had irrevocably damaged her lungs, making her prey to a variety of serious diseases. She became one of the unlucky 15 to 20 percent of smokers who develop COPD. In fact, she should count herself fortunate that she doesn't have any of the other heart or lung diseases caused by smoking — lung cancer being the leading one. In 1995, more than 17,000 Canadians died from lung cancer; approximately 85 percent of lung cancer cases are a direct result of cigarette smoking.

"Lungs Are for Life" — this slogan of The Lung Association says it all. Our lungs are built to last without ever letting us down — if they stay healthy. We can even lead a normal, active life with only one lung, as long as it's healthy. Our lungs age as we grow older, but they remain strong enough that even the lungs of a hundred-year-old can still support a normal life. On the other hand, because our lungs are so vital for a healthy body, when lung disease does strike, the consequences are usually serious.

That delicate, complicated respiratory system we talked about in chapter 1 can be easily, and irreversibly, messed up. Smoking is one of the easiest ways to do that. But there are many other causes of lung disease, ranging from air pollution to infections to genetic defects to drug abuse. You've probably heard of some of the other common diseases that affect the lungs: cystic fibrosis, tuberculosis, pneumonia, asthma, farmer's lung. Some are less well known — sarcoidosis and bronchiectasis, for example. In chapter 15, we'll take a quick look at these other lung diseases, but for now let's concentrate on COPD.

Obstructive and Restrictive Lung Diseases

Lung diseases are divided into two basic categories: **obstructive** and **restrictive**.

Obstructive lung diseases, like COPD, affect the breathing passages, or airways. As the name implies, these passageways become obstructed, making it difficult to get air out of, and sometimes into, the lungs. Obstructive diseases tend to have their main impact on exhaling air from the lungs — breathing out. When we expand our chests to inhale, the volume of the chest cavity increases, causing the airways to expand, or dilate, a bit to make it easier to breathe in. When we breathe out, the chest cavity relaxes and gets smaller as the air leaves, so the airways close down slightly and become narrower.

Air usually has no problem getting out of the lungs — it is pushed out as the elastic lungs and chest wall contract. However, when diseases such as asthma or COPD constrict the airways, it becomes more difficult to breathe out easily. Also, because the airways are obstructed, the flow of air becomes **turbulent**, like water from a lake trying to exit via a narrow stream. Turbulent airflow makes noise; we call this **wheezing**. Disease causes obstruction to the airways in several ways, but the bottom line is that breathing out becomes much more difficult, and this leads to breathlessness.

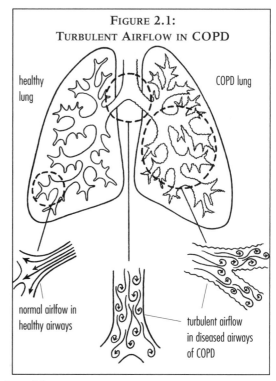

FIGURE 2.1:
TURBULENT AIRFLOW IN COPD

healthy lung

COPD lung

normal airlfow in healthy airways

turbulent airflow in diseased airways of COPD

With advanced airway obstruction, it becomes really difficult to breathe out all the air you've just breathed in. Some stays behind, keeping the lungs overfilled or **hyperinflated**. Try this on yourself to simulate the effect. Take in a deep breath but don't exhale. Take in another and another. You're hyperinflated. Hold it! Now run upstairs. You'll soon appreciate what it feels like to have COPD or asthma.

Figure 2.2 shows the chest X-rays of two people — one is normal, the other, with COPD, is hyperinflated.

Restrictive lung diseases, on the other hand, prevent the lungs or the chest from expanding fully to take in a breath. It's like wearing a too-tight corset — it's hard to breathe in. Restriction can result from disease of the lung tissue itself, the outer lining of the lungs (the **pleura**), or the chest wall. When the lung tissue (the spongy part of the lungs) becomes scarred, or fibrosed, by disease, it can no longer expand or contract easily: it's restricted. Think of a soft, damp sponge that's become hard and dried out. If the pleura becomes thickened or scarred, it can no longer stretch

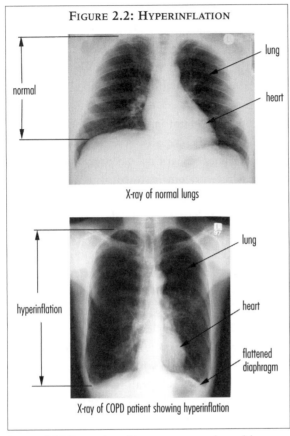

FIGURE 2.2: HYPERINFLATION

normal

lung

heart

X-ray of normal lungs

hyperinflation

lung

heart

flattened diaphragm

X-ray of COPD patient showing hyperinflation

easily; as a result, it prevents the underlying lung from expanding easily with each breath.

The same can happen if the chest wall (the ribs, muscles, and abdomen) becomes stiff with disease — arthritis, for example. The most common cause of chest wall restriction is a "big gut." Abdominal obesity makes it difficult for your lungs to expand when you breathe because you have to work so hard to move your belly out of the way. If you have COPD *and* a big gut, your breathlessness may be particularly troublesome because you're suffering from both an obstructive and a restrictive problem.

Since people with restrictive diseases of the lungs can take in only shallow breaths, they tend to breathe more rapidly than healthy people. Patients with restrictive diseases have difficulty breathing in, but breathing out is usually easy for them.

Chronic Obstructive Pulmonary Disease

Don wheezes, coughs, and spits. Janet finds herself short of breath when performing the simplest household tasks. Mychelle, like Don, has a smoker's cough but she's still able to keep active, golfing up to five times each week in the summer, downhill skiing a couple of days each week in the winter. Louise would love to be like Mychelle, but she's tethered to an oxygen tank because the level of oxygen in her blood is too low. Arthur putters in his garden all summer long, but his yard is off limits in the winter because he can't catch his breath in the cold. For Jean, it's the hot, humid weather that affects her breathing. She hibernates in her air-conditioned condo when summer days get too sweltering.

All these people are different. Their symptoms vary. And their tolerance for their symptoms varies also. But they've all got COPD. As you will learn, COPD is a disease with lots of variations and degrees of severity. A new definition of COPD was recently put forward by a World Health Organization group called Global Initiative for Chronic Obstructive Lung Disease (GOLD) that aims to promote better worldwide care and research for COPD. Here is their simple definition: "COPD is a disease characterized by a progressive airflow obstruction caused by an abnormal inflammatory reaction to the chronic inhalation of noxious particles." Let's see what this really means.

We've talked about how the normal lung works and how the delicate respiratory system can be easily damaged, particularly by cigarette smoking. We know smoking ("the chronic inhalation of noxious particles") is the primary cause of COPD, but what precisely is this disease?

Chronic obstructive pulmonary disease is a grab-bag term. It includes two major breathing disorders: chronic bronchitis and emphysema. Since both disorders are caused by cigarette smoking, they tend to coexist in COPD patients. Chronic bronchitis and emphysema lead to breathlessness and an accelerated decline in lung function with age as well. So even though the term emphysema is often used as if it were a synonym for COPD, you'd be hard pressed to find a COPD patient who is suffering exclusively from either chronic bronchitis or emphysema alone.

Take Audrey, for example. Her days are partly spent coughing and clearing excessive mucus from her lungs and airways, which is a certain sign that she has chronic bronchitis, the "cough and spit" component of COPD. But if you perform a specialized lung function test on Audrey, or look at her lungs with a specialized X-ray called a CT scan, you would see that her lungs have large holes in them. That means she has emphysema too.

Here's where it can get confusing. Many terms are used to describe obstructive diseases of the lungs: asthma, COPD, chronic bronchitis, emphysema, bronchiectasis, COLD (chronic obstructive lung disease), CAL (chronic airflow limitation), and CAO (chronic airflow obstruction), to name just a few. Doctors, nurses, and respiratory therapists don't always use these terms in the same way. In the worst-case scenario, some patients who truly have COPD with emphysema (holes in the lungs) predominating may be told that they have bad asthma (airway inflammation and spasm, but no lung holes). Furthermore, if the diagnosis is not precise, the doctor may tend to push asthma therapy on the patient. However, asthma therapy often does not help patients with emphysema, and may distract the doctor away from therapies that could be of greater benefit. On the other hand, it's not uncommon for an asthmatic who also happens to be a long-term smoker to be misidentified as having COPD or emphysema.

To be fair, without specialized tests it's not always easy to sort out the differences among asthma, chronic bronchitis, and emphysema or to tell whether these conditions coexist in the same patient. The symptoms of various obstructive lung diseases are often very similar. COPD and asthma, for example, are often characterized by a similar constellation of symptoms, including

— shortness of breath (**dyspnea** is the technical term),
— chronic cough,
— increased production of phlegm, and
— fatigue.

Take a look at two people with COPD. Don suffers primarily from chronic bronchitis. He's plagued by coughing and spitting. Sometimes he is short of breath — when he's out walking, for example — but he lists coughing as his primary symptom. For Janet, it's breathlessness. "Picture yourself with a drinking straw," she says. "One end is in your mouth, your finger is blocking the other end. You try to suck in some air. Of course, you get nothing. When my breathing feels like this, I know I'm getting into trouble. I feel that, if I could get my hand inside my chest and push out whatever it is that's obstructing my breathing, I'd be okay." Janet will often find herself short of breath with the slightest exertion. She's troubled by coughing only periodically. She suffers primarily from emphysema but she has elements of chronic bronchitis as well.

21

But Janet and Don share one major problem: like everyone who has COPD, they are afflicted by "chronic airflow obstruction," which progresses slowly over time and is, for the most part, irreversible. Translation: exhaling is a problem for all who suffer from COPD. You can't empty your lungs as easily or completely as a person with healthy lungs. As the name says, chronic obstructive pulmonary disease is a disorder of the lungs that is ongoing and characterized by an obstruction or blockage to the flow of air into and out of the lungs. And, once you've got it, you'll always have it — it won't go away. The true challenges of COPD are prevention, stabilization, and management of the disease, including flare-ups.

Although Don and Janet both suffer from airflow obstruction, an examination of their lungs would reveal different degrees of pathology (illness) and different reasons for the obstruction. But there's often very little difference in the way chronic bronchitis and emphysema are treated. And that helps explain why they're usually lumped together under the banner of COPD.

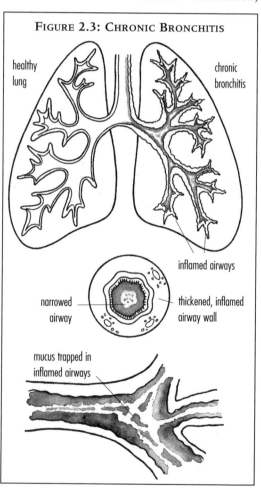

FIGURE 2.3: CHRONIC BRONCHITIS

healthy lung

chronic bronchitis

inflamed airways

narrowed airway

thickened, inflamed airway wall

mucus trapped in inflamed airways

Chronic Bronchitis

You can hear Don from down the hall and around the corner. He's coughing. You'd probably call it a smoker's cough: loud coughs are coming from deep inside his lungs. And you know that at the end of it, Don will have to spit out some phlegm. It's what doctors call a **productive cough**.

Apart from the coughing and spitting, Don considers himself a pretty healthy person. "My lungs," he says, "are like the bilge pump on my boat. They start working when they want to and the phlegm just comes right up. I don't have much control over it. It's quite embarrassing at times. And the volume is amazing — much more now than when I first started testing for COPD. Let me tell you, I carry a good supply of tissue with me at all times."

Chronic bronchitis is the predominant form of COPD affecting Don. The name says it all. It's an inflammation and weeping of the bronchial tubes (bronchitis) that won't go away (chronic). The term chronic obstructive bronchitis is also used, emphasizing the airflow obstruction that characterizes this condition.

Chronic bronchitis must be distinguished from **acute bronchitis**, a condition most people have had at one time or another. Acute bronchitis is a short-lived inflammation of the bronchial tubes, usually due to a viral infection — in other words, a chest cold that eventually goes away. Chronic bronchitis, on the other hand, does not go away.

Constant exposure to cigarette smoke, air pollution, and even chronic or repeated airway infections in young life can lead to the changes we see in the airways of those with chronic bronchitis. Like many people with chronic bronchitis, Don experienced lung problems during his childhood. "I had pneumonia half a dozen times when I was a kid, plus other things like bronchitis." For Don, however, like the vast majority of other patients, cigarette smoking was the main culprit.

The changes in the airways caused by chronic bronchitis consist of inflammation of the airway walls accompanied by an enlargement and overgrowth of the bronchial mucous glands, usually due to the chronic irritation of years of inhaling cigarette smoke with all its toxins. These changes lead to an overproduction of mucus in the airways. The mucus tends to be thick and therefore difficult to clear from the tubes. Clearing the tubes is made even more difficult because cigarette smoke also destroys the cilia on the epithelial cells lining the airways. Because of the damaged cilia, the extra mucus can't be moved very easily, forcing you to cough frequently to clear your airways.

Under the stimulus of chronic mucus production, nerve receptors in the bronchial tubes begin sending messages to the brain: "Too much mucus down here. It's starting to narrow the airways and it's making breathing difficult. Do something!" The brain responds and you start coughing. If the cough works as it should, you'll start emptying your lungs of some of the excess mucus. That's the phlegm you spit out.

Not only do people with chronic bronchitis cough constantly, but they are also breathless with the exertion. That's partly because their airways are swollen and partially blocked by mucus, making it harder for air to move in and out of the lungs easily, and partly because they usually have an element of emphysema too. The result is that people like Don have to work hard to breathe, and this causes breathlessness and eventually fatigue.

Emphysema

Watch Janet talk and you're watching her fight for every breath. Each year for the past decade, she has found her activities slightly more limited by her shortness of breath. In 1999, she gave up shovelling snow from her driveway; soon she expects to stop washing her car. She's still able to vacuum the house, however, as long as she paces herself and carefully plans her route around each floor.

Breathlessness dominates Janet's life. It's there constantly, and that's typical of someone whose COPD is mainly emphysema. There's not much active chronic bronchitis in her lungs. She doesn't cough up much phlegm anymore. A CT scan of her lungs would show the characteristic thinning of her lung tissue into wispy strands and a profusion of wide open spaces — the holes in the lungs that result from cigarette-

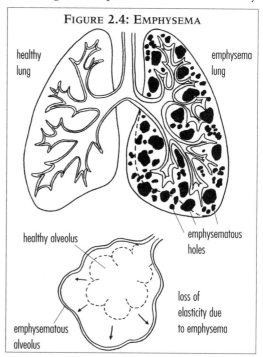

FIGURE 2.4: EMPHYSEMA

healthy lung

emphysema lung

healthy alveolus

emphysematous holes

loss of elasticity due to emphysema

emphysematous alveolus

induced destruction of normal tissue. (For a representative CT scan of emphysema, see Figure 4.5 in chapter 4.)

How does emphysema occur? In everyone's lungs, certain cells in the airways release an enzyme called **protease** that is helpful in combating bacterial infection. However, if too much protease is released, it can act to digest lung tissue, leaving destructive holes unless the protease is

CAUSES OF COPD

In North America cigarette smoking is the most commonly recognized cause of COPD — both chronic bronchitis and emphysema. However, despite significant smoking histories, only about 15 to 20 percent of smokers seem to develop COPD. This suggests to medical researchers that genetic factors, as yet undefined and undiscovered, probably confer a high risk for susceptibility to the effects of cigarette smoking for some people. In other words, if you possess the genetic risk factors for COPD, your odds of contracting COPD are much greater than those of a smoker who doesn't. It is also thought that there are genetic determinants for addiction to nicotine.

In countries less developed than Canada and the United States, chronic or recurrent infections of the airways beginning in childhood are more common and likely lead to destructive changes in the lungs that can result in COPD for some individuals.

Air pollution is recognized as a trigger for flare-ups of established COPD, and may also exert a synergistic effect with cigarette smoking in causing COPD, although this link has been difficult to prove.

Some occupations associated with chronic exposure to certain dusts and chemicals (e.g., cotton dust and certain ingredients in plastics and adhesives called isocyanates) may contribute to the development of COPD.

A familial association of COPD has been demonstrated. Children of smoking parents are more likely to develop COPD and asthma, for example. However, these same children are also more likely to be cigarette smokers themselves. It has been difficult to clearly demonstrate that chronic exposure to smoke from other smokers (passive smoking or second-hand smoke) can contribute to the development of COPD, although this is likely to occur, at least for those high-risk individuals who have a genetic disposition to the disease.

A rare genetic deficiency of the anti-protease alpha$_1$-antitrypsin is associated with the development of emphysema at an early age (thirty to forty years old). The disease probably results from the unopposed action of naturally occurring protease in the lung, leading to tissue destruction and eventual early-onset emphysema. Cigarette smoking naturally worsens the situation. This genetic deficiency is very rare, accounting for only one in 6,000 people in the general population, and less than 1 percent of all COPD in North America.

Alpha$_1$-antitrypsin deficiency can be detected with a simple blood test and should be suspected in anyone with emphysema who has a minimal smoking history or is under the age of forty-five, and in anyone who has a family history of premature COPD. Replacement therapy with alpha$_1$-antitrypsin is possible, but it is very expensive and, to date, has not been shown to alter the eventual progression of emphysema, although research is continuing.

neutralized. To protect our lungs from this "auto-digestion," we all have chemicals called **protease inhibitors** that block protease and prevent lung destruction and the development of emphysema.

Emphysema develops if the protease increases in amount or if the anti-protease activity is diminished, or both. Smokers who develop emphysema do so because of the double-whammy effect of cigarette smoke: not only does smoking increase the amount of protease by stimulating the cells that produce the enzyme but it also blocks the effect of the anti-protease, leaving the protease auto-digestion to run amok. The result is lungs that resemble Swiss cheese. Although there is a very rare form of emphysema caused by a genetic defect in the amount of anti-protease produced, the vast majority of emphysema, at least in industrialized countries like Canada and the United States, is due to the effects of cigarette smoke.

People with predominantly emphysema have a constant struggle with breathlessness, yet they don't have that much chronic bronchitis. Breathlessness from emphysema can have several causes, but by far the main culprit is hyperinflation of the lungs. (The term emphysema comes from the Greek for puffed up.)

HYPERINFLATION — WHAT CAUSES IT?

Hyperinflation means exactly what it sounds like: too much air gets trapped in the lungs, like an over-inflated balloon. There are two main reasons for this:

1. Emphysematous airways tend to narrow excessively, often collapsing when you try to exhale, because the unchecked auto-digestion of the elastic fibres in the airways leaves them soft, "wimpy," and easily compressed. When you try to exhale forcefully, the pressure inside your chest cavity increases. With healthy lungs, the airways are strong enough to stay open and the pressure of a forced exhalation helps to push air out of the lungs normally. With emphysematous airways, however, the pressure of a forced exhalation causes the non-elastic airways to collapse. Air can't leave the lungs and remains trapped inside. Technically, this is called **dynamic hyperinflation**.

2. The unchecked protease enzymes thin out and weaken the lung tissue itself. It's as if a thick, industrial-strength balloon that is very elastic and deflates rapidly has been replaced by an old, thinned-out balloon that can barely empty itself. Remember, at the end of a natural breath in, the lungs are filled with air and thus stretched. When you relax your breathing muscles to let the air out of your lungs, the stretched lungs contract (like a balloon releasing its air) and the air is pushed out from the lungs. If you have emphysema, the lungs can no longer contract forcefully and the inhaled air is not completely exhaled. The net result is hyperinflated lungs (look back at figure 2.2)

Why does that make you breathless? Remember our experiment? Breathe in until your lungs are full to bursting. Hold it for a while. It's not comfortable and you're starting to feel breathless. Run upstairs. You're really breathless now. People with severe emphysema walk around hyperinflated like this all the time. No wonder Janet is always short of breath.

Interestingly, although COPD makes it difficult to breathe air out of the lungs easily, most people with advanced COPD associate their breathlessness with an inability to get enough air into the lungs. The reason? Hyperinflation. When the lungs are hyperinflated because of COPD, you have to work extra hard to get more air *into* the lungs with each breath. This extra work results in horrible breathlessness. (Technically speaking, severe hyperinflation due to airflow obstruction is also a restrictive process, because hyperinflation prevents further chest expansion.)

Of course, there's more to it than hyperinflation and an inability to empty the lungs normally. If your lungs are always hyperinflated, where is the room for your next breath of air? With hyperinflation, the main breathing muscle, the diaphragm, is chronically stretched flat. As a result, the diaphragm has no more room to contract and move downward to help bring in that next breath of air. In this circumstance, the only way to move air into the lungs is to call upon the **supplementary muscles**, or **accessory muscles**, of breathing to help out.

The accessory muscles are mainly the muscles you can feel at the side of your neck when you breathe forcefully (see Figure 1.3). Healthy people without COPD use these muscles all the time — but only when they're exercising. If you have COPD and significant hyperinflation, however, you'll need to use these muscles even when you're at rest. This means you have to do more muscular work to breathe. That in turn causes more breathlessness and more fatigue. It's as if a person with emphysema is exercising all the time. It's tiring. Just ask Janet!

Oxygen Alert! Pay Attention to Your Oxygen Levels

Other factors besides hyperinflation can make you breathless if you have COPD. For example, advanced COPD can lead to a low blood oxygen level, called **hypoxemia**. Hypoxemia stimulates you to try to breathe more deeply and rapidly in an attempt to get more oxygen. But with COPD, this increased drive to breathe only makes you work harder, since it's difficult to move air in and out of the lungs easily. And more breathing work means more breathlessness.

Advanced emphysema contributes to hypoxemia because of the Swiss cheese effect. The destructive process of emphysema greatly reduces the amount of lung tissue available for oxygen exchange. When the surface area of your lungs is reduced from the size of a tennis court to the size of a couple of ping-pong tables (about 25 percent of normal), you can have problems getting enough oxygen into your system.

Chronic bronchitis can also contribute to low blood oxygen and breathlessness. When your airways are swollen, inflamed, and clogged with mucus, it is difficult for oxygen to make it through the airways and into your blood. Similarly, the waste gas — carbon dioxide — can't make it out of the airways easily.

When the level of oxygen in your blood falls below a critical value, you'll begin to feel breathless. An inadequate supply of oxygen means that there isn't enough reaching the tissues of the body. This lack of oxygen makes every part of you function poorly. You'll feel breathless, very tired, and mentally sluggish.

A sign that your blood oxygen levels might be dangerously low is a bluish discoloration of your tongue and the inside of your lips. The outside of the lips, the nail beds, and the skin may also look blue. This is called **cyanosis**. We've all had cyanosis of our fingers, toes, and lips at one time or another. Think of the child emerging from a cold lake with chattering teeth and blue lips and nails. In that case, cyanosis is a sign that the child is cold — the blood vessels in the lips and fingers have clamped down to reduce heat loss. The cyanosis disappears as soon as the child warms up. If you're not cold, however, and you notice cyanosis of your lips, tongue, fingers, or skin that doesn't fade, you may have low blood oxygen or heart failure. You should be checked by your doctor.

Swelling (**edema**) of your ankles may be another warning sign that your blood oxygen levels are dangerously low. The swelling may build up over time as your COPD worsens and your blood oxygen levels fall. When the blood oxygen level falls below that critical threshold, it causes the blood vessels in the lungs to constrict somewhat. This can lead to a form of high blood pressure within the arteries of the lungs called **pulmonary hypertension**. This high blood pressure may be restricted only to your lungs. The blood pressure usually measured in your arm may be completely normal.

Pulmonary hypertension puts a strain on the chambers of the right side of the heart. This, combined with an effect on the kidneys due to low blood oxygen, causes your body to retain fluids. Eventually, this produces puffy ankles. There can be other causes of puffy ankles, such as poor circulation in the legs, arthritis, and hardening of the arteries around the heart. But if you have COPD and you begin to notice puffy ankles or legs, ask your doctor to check your blood oxygen level. You may need additional therapy for COPD, or even to start breathing supplemental oxygen in your home. Home oxygen therapy will increase the oxygen level in your blood and thus reduce the high blood pressure in the lungs, which in turn takes the strain off the heart, reducing the stimulus for swollen ankles and legs. Pulmonary hypertension can also contribute to breathlessness, especially with exertion, because of the added strain it puts on the heart. That is another reason why breathing supplemental oxygen may help reduce breathlessness in certain cases.

(*Don't be complacent if you notice that your puffy ankles disappear overnight. The extra fluid is still there; it's just shifted to your back and abdomen while you were lying down. Chances are your puffy ankles will be back by afternoon.*)

Oxygen therapy may not relieve breathlessness completely. Breathing supplemental oxygen only corrects those causes of breathlessness associated with hypoxemia. All the other causes of breathlessness (the swollen, clogged airways, the airway narrowing, the hyperinflation, and the strain on the breathing muscles) still remain, despite oxygen therapy. Chapter 11 provides more details on home oxygen.

3

The Preventative Maintenance Plan — The Key to Coping with COPD

"*M*y first thought when the doctor told me I had COPD was 'I have to get better,'" says Peg. "I assumed there was a wonder drug that would cure me. It was a bitter pill to swallow to learn I was never going to rid myself of COPD. I prayed to God I wouldn't get any worse. But prayers, I learned, are not enough. I needed to work at stabilizing my disease — I needed to learn about COPD, change my lifestyle, and find professionals to help me. And I could never go back to cigarettes."

COPD is a disease and, as with all diseases, both patients and physicians often tend to hope they can alter its progression with drugs alone. Unfortunately, COPD is a chronic illness with no easy treatment. Unless there is a significant asthmatic component, the airflow obstruction associated with COPD tends not to respond dramatically to drug therapy. (Drug therapy for COPD is discussed in detail in chapter 10.)

There are, however, many ways other than drugs to manage this difficult disease. Drug therapy is only one element in a comprehensive management plan for COPD. Research has shown that exercise, good nutrition, and an understanding of the disease help patients learn to live and cope with COPD. And that's what the majority of this book is about.

We'll look at the big picture, and tell you how to suspect whether you might have COPD, how COPD is diagnosed, and, most important, how to develop a preventative maintenance plan tailored to you and your disease.

Your plan suit your needs, your life, and your abilities. Each person's approach to managing COPD will be different, depending on individual elements in his or her preventative maintenance plan. Look at our group, for example: Audrey and Mychelle are exercise addicts; Raymond and Janet work diligently on healthy eating; Peg and Don have found new ways to keep themselves mentally active. They may be doing things differently from one another, but they all have a lot in common. They've spent time thinking about their disease, setting long-term goals for themselves, and working to achieve those goals. They've all come to the difficult realization that there's no cure for this thing. How they plan to live the rest of their lives with COPD is in their hands.

Like them, you too can work out the elements of your comprehensive management plan. But first, you need to take a look at the big picture, which is all of the elements that go into the development of a complete preventative maintenance plan. Here's a quick checklist to get you thinking. You'll find a full discussion of each element in the chapters that follow.

1. **Diagnosing COPD.** How can you tell whether you have COPD? The first step in managing COPD is to be sure of the diagnosis. You should suspect you might have COPD if you are a current or past smoker (even a "light" smoker) and are experiencing troublesome cough, phlegm, or breathlessness. Maybe you think you're just getting old or out of shape, but maybe not — these symptoms may be early-warning signs that your lungs are not healthy. You should see your doctor and ask the simple question "Could I have COPD?" If COPD is a possibility, your doctor should arrange for you to have a breathing test called **spirometry**. This test (explained in chapter 4) is crucial for an accurate diagnosis of COPD. If the spirometry test is not offered and you are still concerned about the possibility of COPD, insist on having it. It may be the most important test you'll take.

2. **Attempting to Alter the Progression of COPD.** We know more about the science of asthma than we do about the science of COPD. In fact, we now have drugs that can alter the progression of asthma by

preventing the development of irreversible damage to the breathing tubes. We may not be able to cure asthma but, in certain situations, we can prevent it from becoming worse. We would like to be able to do the same thing for COPD but, at this time, we simply don't understand enough about the workings of the disease to have developed suitable drugs. However, we do have drugs to control the symptoms of COPD, and these are discussed in chapter 10.

Don't be discouraged. There are many other things we can do to help. The best strategy we currently have for prevention in COPD is smoking cessation (or not starting in the first place). We know that COPD patients run the risk of worsening their condition by

PEG

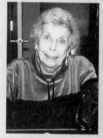

"Give me a minute." That's Peg's favourite saying. She'll say those words a dozen times each day to her husband when he calls her to the breakfast table, to a store clerk who wants her to walk across a store, to her friends when they ask her to join them for coffee. "I've got to have that minute to catch my breath," explains Peg. "I've learned that if I launch into things without catching my breath, my breathing will get out of control and I'll panic. So instead of getting caught up in it, I sit back, stop what I'm doing, and wait a bit. It's just one of the many lessons I've learned during the eight years I've lived with this disease."

At seventy-five, Peg is a very active woman. Politics keep her busy these days. She's the deputy reeve of the rural township she moved to when she retired. Several evenings each month, she's out at meetings.

COPD came as a great shock for Peg. "I raised four children, worked as a comptroller for a grocer and real estate company. I also took courses at university and loved to cross-country ski. I was active the whole time I was raising kids and I was never out of breath," she recalls. "I just couldn't believe that I would ever be short of breath. That could happen to somebody else but not me. I refused to even say the word 'emphysema' — it's such an ugly word. To me, it meant old gasping men with oxygen tanks."

These attitudes spelled trouble for Peg. After her diagnosis, she could not and would not accept that she had COPD. This denial led her to spurn treatment. She refused to attend rehabilitation programs. "It was a long time before I could accept that I had COPD. And I don't think I'm fully there even now," she comments.

Peg acknowledges that she was both propelled and held back by her own personality — her pride, in particular. She's an independent, stubborn woman; an achiever. She did not want anyone's pity. She found it difficult to start relying on her husband, Harold, for support. "I never want people feeling sorry for *me* and I certainly did not want anyone to see me gasping for air!" In fact, when she was first continuing to smoke. Their lung function will decline much more rapidly as they age if they persist in smoking. Smoking cessation is critical. And it's never too late to butt out. We'll talk more about this important topic in chapter 9.

3. **Preventing Complications of COPD.** The goal is to limit flare-ups of your COPD and avoid hospitalizations. COPD patients are more susceptible than healthy people to damaging lung infections. Lung infections in COPD can produce serious complications that can lead to additional lung damage. Because this damage can accumulate over the years, patients should attempt to avoid lung infections and, if one does develop, seek early treatment to prevent further damage.

diagnosed with COPD, she didn't even tell her four children.

So what changed for Peg? Reality hit her square in the face. She couldn't control her breathing and she'd panic ("The kind of panic where you think your next breath is your last"). Then she'd be begging Harold to take her to the emergency department, where she'd be given bronchodilator medication. After several such incidents, she realized she needed help. Her respirologist arranged a six-week stay at a local rehabilitation centre.

"Rehabilitation saved my life," Peg says. "They taught me that I wasn't sick, that I wasn't going to die, and that I was a perfectly good person. I worked with respiratory therapists, occupational therapists, psychologists. I exercised every day. I finally realized what I had and decided I wanted to stabilize my condition. I began to conquer my fear of COPD by learning little tricks that helped me keep my breathing under control."

But Peg faced another difficult hurdle in 1996, when her respiratory therapist suggested she start using a walker. "For me, a walker was a sign of weakness. I wanted to get better, not worse. It was a really hard decision to start using it." It made her private disease public. But, being the practical woman she is, Peg knew she had a choice to make. Sit at home without a walker or be able to travel with one. She's come to treasure her walker. It's what makes it possible for her to travel to Atlantic City with friends and allows her to shop with her daughter. It's what keeps her active.

Peg knows she's not all the way there in her acceptance of COPD. She still finds it very difficult to speak openly and honestly to her friends about how she's feeling. She acknowledges that she doesn't want to appear to be a complainer. "I always say I'm fine when they ask me," she says. "That means there are certain things I won't do with them because I don't want them to see me struggling."

Peg has a recurring dream. In her dream, she's running, quickly, gracefully, and easily. She is running alongside her children. "I know I can't do that. I'm sure that's the reason I have that dream. It's because I want to do it so badly." She knows that ability will not return. "COPD has changed my life," she says. "And I've learned that because of COPD, I must continue to adapt if I want to stay active. And I will stay active." Even if that means using a walker.

It's recommended that all COPD patients receive an annual influenza vaccination. A pneumonia vaccination, given only once in a lifetime, is also recommended. We'll talk about managing flare-ups and lung infections in chapter 14.

Vaccinations are one way of warding off lung infections. Staying healthy is another. Preventing the weakening of not just the breathing muscles but the body in general is an excellent strategy to help you better cope with COPD. Eating nutritiously (gaining or losing weight, if necessary), getting enough exercise to maintain physical fitness, and avoiding debilitating habits such as drinking too much alcohol are also excellent goals. Professionals call this "pulmonary rehabilitation," and we discuss how you can get started on your "rehab" in chapter 7.

4. **Getting Help When You Need It.** It all sounds pretty easy when the instructions are listed in a couple of sentences — avoid lung infections, strengthen your breathing muscles, eat nutritiously — but all of these tasks are hard work when you're not feeling well. That means you'll need help and support to achieve these goals. Get help from family and friends, and make sure you know how to locate the professional help you need from doctors, respiratory therapists, pharmacists, and others who can work with you. Education is another integral component of your plan. Learning the details of what you need and why, together with knowledge of how to accomplish your goals, will help you stay healthy and strong. All these issues are discussed in chapters 5 and 6.

5. **Controlling the Symptoms of COPD.** Since we don't have drugs that can predictably alter the natural history of COPD, the main goal of drug therapy is to reduce the symptoms of breathlessness, cough, phlegm, and fatigue that accompany the disease. We use bronchodilators and theophyllines to reduce the work of breathing for COPD patients; inhaled corticosteroids are sometimes used to reduce cough and inflammation. The response to these drugs, however, is much less dramatic for the COPD patient than for the asthmatic. We'll talk more about how to get the most out of drug therapy for COPD in chapter 10.

Oxygen is also considered a drug. It can be very helpful for improving breathlessness and exercise tolerance in patients who have an abnormally low concentration of oxygen in their blood, a condition called hypoxemia. Oxygen therapy may also help improve longevity for COPD patients. It is discussed in detail in chapter 11.

Physical fitness, together with the maintenance of an ideal weight and healthy eating habits, is another key ingredient for controlling symptoms of COPD. Patients who become out of shape and malnourished run the risk of increased breathlessness, cough, and phlegm. With those symptoms come anxiety and panic. To avoid this vicious cycle, you want to be as healthy and physically active as your lungs will allow. Tips on how to gently "get off your butt" are presented in chapter 8. Of course, the very best thing you can do for yourself is to "butt out" and "get off your butt"!

6. **Relearning the Enjoyment of Life — Despite COPD.** Life is not only about fitness and nutrition. You want to live a full life that might include visits with your family, travelling, work, volunteer activities, hobbies — you name it. Your plan should also include attention to the quality of your life. Depression, anger, guilt, and fear, for example, are common companions of COPD, and medical help is available for all of them. Coping strategies that help you do your housework, keep up with your friends, stay busy in the community, and prepare meals — to name just a few of your many activities — can be more important to you and your health than the drugs you take for your COPD. And many patients can achieve a natural and fulfilling sex life. All of these issues are crucial elements of your preventative maintenance plan and we'll talk about them in chapters 6, 8, 12, and 13.

7. **Planning for the Future.** COPD is both chronic and incurable. It will prematurely end the life of some people. Your plans for the future should take into consideration the presence of COPD in your life. End-of-life decision making is a difficult subject to think about and discuss, but it's something all people with COPD should incorporate into their COPD management plan. We help with this emotional subject in chapter 14.

The Big Picture

In an ideal world, every person with COPD would try to accomplish each and every element of a comprehensive preventative maintenance plan. We don't, however, live in an ideal world. But by reading this book you are taking an important step right now. In the remaining pages, you'll learn more about your disease, how it is diagnosed and followed, the possible treatments, and how other people have dealt with their disease. Learning about your options — and their benefits and drawbacks — is your first step toward taking control of your COPD. Once you've seen the "big picture," the next steps are up to you!

4

"I Think You'll Need Some Tests"
— Diagnosing COPD

Read this chapter even if you've already been diagnosed with COPD! Because COPD is a chronic condition, you'll be living with it for the rest of your life. Unlike diagnosing a broken leg or a bout of pneumonia, the diagnostic process for a COPD patient is not a one-shot deal. As you age, for example, your COPD will change and new elements of the disease or complications will be diagnosed by your doctor. Knowing something about the procedures and tests used for diagnosing and monitoring your COPD will help you get the most out of this ongoing process of assessment and reassessment.

When you read the profiles of our group of COPD patients, you'll see that some of them felt that COPD came upon them like a shot out of the blue. Louise, for example, was a busy nurse, logging sixteen-hour shifts. She thought she was an extremely healthy woman until she was struck down by a bout of the flu during the winter of 1996. She landed in the intensive care unit suffering from respiratory failure. It was during that hospitalization that she was diagnosed with COPD. It seemed to her that she'd gone from health to disability overnight.

Now that Louise knows more about COPD, she realizes that the disease had been with her for many years before her dramatic hospitalization. She'd long suffered from a smoker's cough. Every cold went straight to her chest, resulting in a bout of acute infective bronchitis and a course of antibiotics. But none of her ailments were ever quite severe enough to make her miss more than a couple of days from work. She didn't think of speaking to her doctor about her breathing, and, even though she was a smoker with a chronic cough, her doctor never discussed the possibility of COPD and never suggested testing her lung function.

Louise didn't know she had a problem with her lungs. She was working and seemed able to do all the things she wanted to do. However, during her hospitalization she realized that over the previous couple of years, she'd started to become very tired during her long nursing shifts. In retrospect, she'd slowed down quite a bit. But she'd cut out activities so gradually that she didn't see the pattern until it was too late. Neither did her doctor.

Louise's story is not uncommon. Her COPD is dominated by emphysema, and the diagnosis of emphysema is often delayed because of its insidious onset. If you're susceptible to the ravages of cigarette smoke, emphysema probably begins with your first pack of cigarettes. The more you smoke, the quicker and more extensive the damage will be. Louise, at a pack or more each day, was a solid, steady smoker. But, in its early stages, emphysema can be a silent disease. Its sufferers often don't display the musical chest, coughing, and spitting that those with chronic bronchitis do. Emphysema slowly and progressively chips away at lung function. Because it proceeds so slowly, sufferers often chalk up their bouts of breathlessness and fatigue to aging. And because they feel they're "just getting old," they don't go to a doctor until they find themselves, like Louise, in a critical and disabled state.

Its quiet approach means that emphysema often goes undiagnosed. But although it's noisier, chronic bronchitis can also be easily ignored in its early stages. Sufferers chalk up their ailments to "just another cold" or "just a smoker's cough." Doctors and smokers alike should be sensitive to the insidious development of COPD. Doctors should regularly measure the lung function of all smokers, regardless of age, to help achieve earlier diagnosis and, ideally, earlier prevention.

Early diagnosis of COPD is essential. With early diagnosis comes the possibility of preventing further damage to the lungs. If smokers listen to entreaties to stop smoking and throw away their cigarettes as soon as they're diagnosed with COPD, they'll have taken the biggest step they can to prevent further deterioration of their lungs. Early referral for lung function testing is the key to early diagnosis of COPD for long-term smokers. COPD is always a possibility for any current or past smoker with a history of heavy smoking over many years. If you fit that bill, consider asking your doctor about the possibility of lung function testing, just to be sure. If your doctor does not seem keen on lung function testing, ask again! It's important to know!

The cynic in the crowd might say: "Who cares whether you're diagnosed with COPD earlier rather than later? Once you've got it, that's it, you're never rid of it." In part, that's correct. COPD is irreversible — you'll always have it. But an early diagnosis can mean an earlier start to efforts at preventing further lung damage (mainly smoking cessation) and thus possibly a healthier and longer life. An early and accurate diagnosis can also be very helpful in distinguishing between COPD and asthma. If asthma is ruled out, you and your doctor won't get caught in the trap of concentrating on the asthma-drug approach to your health and instead can focus on drugs that work better in COPD or work on a more useful non-drug approach to COPD management.

Mychelle's experience with COPD diagnosis was similar to Louise's. Like Louise, she didn't suspect she had a lung disease. Naturally, her family doctor had been after her for many years to quit smoking. During one of her regular checkups, he examined her breathing carefully and told her that he suspected COPD. Her COPD was still in its early stages. Although it was tough for her, she gave up smoking within two years of the diagnosis. Her bouts of breathlessness caused her to give up tennis, but she replaced that sport with golf. Knowing that golf wouldn't allow her to keep up the endurance level she could maintain with tennis, and knowing that breathing is an endurance sport, she augmented her fitness regimen with workouts on the treadmill and stationary bike.

If Mychelle hadn't been diagnosed early, she feels she probably would have continued smoking. And she probably wouldn't have worked as diligently at maintaining her fitness level. The diagnosis gave her the impetus she needed to kick the smoking habit and keep exercising. Taken together, these two initiatives have improved her overall prognosis. And this all happened because of an early diagnosis.

Assessment and Reassessment — The Continuing Diagnostic Process

Understanding the diagnostic process continues to be important even after the diagnosis of COPD has been made. Although COPD will never go away, its impact on you and the symptoms it causes will definitely change over the course of your life with the disease. Additional complications of COPD, together with other complications of smoking, including lung cancer and heart disease, can also occur. You must be constantly vigilant, paying attention to your body and learning what you need to do to

MYCHELLE

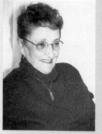

"If someone asks, I tell them I'm in perfect health except . . . Then I explain about my COPD," says Mychelle. "I'm seventy-four years old and this is the only thing wrong with me. So, I'm sort of proud in a way."

She is a woman who knows how to enjoy life, how to find activities that fulfill and suit her tastes, how to love her children. A widow since 1988, she relishes the past but doesn't dwell on her losses. She is intensely close to her five sons, four of whom live nearby and drop in regularly. She eagerly anticipates the future, continually on the lookout for new experiences to tackle. "I've always had a curious nature. I wanted to try everything. And I still do," she exclaims. "I really like to keep up-to-date. I like to know what's going on in the worlds of business, finance, and politics. That's what keeps you young."

Mychelle was born to be busy. As a child, she loved sports, particularly swimming, skiing, and cycling. She married young and gave birth to her sons in quick succession. But she still found time to indulge her passion for sports — skiing at hills throughout Quebec and cycling for miles on end. "When going up a particularly strenuous hill, I'd stop and smoke a cigarette," she recalls.

"I don't hate myself for smoking. I just wish I hadn't started, but I did. I enjoyed it and it affected me badly. That's that," she states. "I was really addicted to cigarettes. Before delivering a baby, I'd be smoking. And right after the baby was born, I'd start again. I felt good in those days. I figured I was one of the people who wouldn't be affected by cigarettes. I still felt immortal. I realize now that I was deluding myself."

Long before she was diagnosed with COPD, Mychelle knew smoking was affecting her health. "My coughing would wake me in the night. I'd tell my husband: 'I'm smoking so much, I'm going to die from it.' It took me ten years to quit smoking. I tried hypnotherapy, laser therapy, listening to records, nicotine gum, the patch. When I was diagnosed with COPD in 1992, I learned that it was an irreversible stabilize your disease and keep your general health as good as it can be. Working with your doctor at each appointment will help you keep on top of your disease and maintain your health.

The diagnostic process is divided into three parts:

— the interview,
— the physical examination, and
— lung function testing.

Together, these elements should provide a definitive and up-to-date diagnosis of your disease and its severity. Get used to all of them because you'll experience them over and over. Remember, if you don't understand any portion of the diagnostic process, ask your doctor for an explanation.

disease and would get worse if I continued to smoke. I just got so fed up with myself that I finally quit cold turkey in 1994."

At one time, all of her sons smoked. Today, only two sons are smokers. It concerns her deeply. But she stops short of telling them what to do. "I was a smoker for so many years and I know how you feel when people tell you what to do. So I send everything I see in magazines and newspapers about COPD to my sons with a note: 'You're not going to like this but I thought you'd be interested in the nature of my illness.' "

Mychelle has given up cycling and put away her tennis racquet. She still skis but ventures out only when the weather suits her. She's replaced the sports she can no longer do with different ones. Golf is now her great love. In the summer months, she plays up to five times each week. On the days when she's short of breath, she uses a golf cart.

Mychelle adamantly refuses to be embarrassed by her condition. "When I'm golfing I often start to cough and need to spit. I try to keep a tissue with me but I sometimes forget. I'll tell my friends: 'I know this isn't appetizing but I'm having a bit of a problem this morning and I've got to spit in the grass.' That's just what I have to do. And, you know what, I've become a very good spitter over the years," she laughs. "I will not feel shy about my COPD."

She's added several new activities to her busy roster — things she can do even if her breathing is bothering her. She plays bridge a couple of times each week. Always a music lover (she worked for many years as an administrator with the University of Ottawa's School of Music), Mychelle attends as many concerts as she can. She's taken up the computer. She's connected to each of her eight grandchildren through email and she's able to correspond with people around the world. Plus, she's become an active volunteer in a niche that suits her physical abilities perfectly: she works for a local museum, transcribing handwritten letters and notes, including a collection of letters written home by soldiers during World War I.

"I may not be able to do all the things I once did. So I'll learn other things," concludes Mychelle.

The Interview

Your doctor will call this part of the process "taking a history." From your perspective, it will probably feel like a job interview. The interview should really be a discussion between you and your doctor, peppered with questions posed by your doctor about you and your health, and questions from you about your health concerns. Your doctor will not be able to diagnose COPD just by talking to you, but a thorough discussion will help the doctor gain a more complete understanding of the impact COPD will have on your life. Information concerning the duration of your cough, whether there is associated phlegm, other medical conditions you might have, your attitude toward medications, and your smoking history provides a rich context against which your doctor will place the results of the tests you will need to undergo, to make a diagnosis of COPD, and to help make decisions about how best to manage your disease.

Here are some of the questions you should expect:

Past history: *Did you have a healthy childhood? Did you have recurring bouts of bronchitis or pneumonia? Did you grow up around smokers? Do you have any allergies?* The answers to questions like these might help your doctor define your risk for having or developing COPD or asthma.

Family history: *Does anyone in your family have asthma, cancer, or heart disease? Does anyone smoke? Does anyone have COPD and, if so, at what age did it come on?* Here the doctor is seeking to define your risk factors for asthma and certain smoking-related diseases, and in particular for the very rare genetic deficiency of alpha$_1$-antitrypsin that is associated with early-onset emphysema.

Smoking: *Do you smoke? Did you smoke in the past? Have you tried quitting? How did you try? Why did you go back to smoking? Do you want to quit now?* A doctor should suspect COPD in anyone and everyone who has a long history of smoking, whether they've quit or not. The doctor will calculate the number of "pack years" you've smoked by dividing the number of cigarettes you smoked each day by twenty (the size of an average pack of smokes) and multiplying that amount by the number of years you've smoked. For example, a forty-cigarette-per-day smoker who's smoked for fifteen years has a pack-year history of thirty years. A twenty-pack-year history is generally considered to indicate an increased risk for the development of COPD, but in reality any regular smoker may be at risk for developing COPD. This quick check of smoking history is important because many COPD patients function for years with no hint that they're developing respiratory problems. Your history of attempts to quit smoking and why you failed (if you did) will help your doctor decide how best to help you quit again — for good!

Working environment: *Have you been exposed to any unusual fumes, dusts, or vapours? Have you worked with chemicals?* Here, your doctor is interested in whether you have been exposed to any toxic substances or certain dusts that may have increased your risk for developing asthma, COPD, or certain other lung diseases, including fibrosis or cancer.

Symptoms: *Do you cough regularly? Is there any phlegm? What colour is it? Is it thick or thin? Have you ever spit blood? Has there been any recent change in your cough or phlegm? Have you ever heard yourself wheeze? Do you have chest pain? Do your ankles swell? Do you get short of breath with exertion? What level of activity (e.g., walking or stair climbing) makes you breathless? Does your breathlessness ever come on spontaneously? Does exposure to anything in particular, such as cat hair or dust, trigger coughing or breathlessness?* Any of these recurring symptoms can be early indicators of lung disease such as asthma, COPD, bronchiectasis, lung cancer, and fibrosis. The new onset of such symptoms may also suggest that a complication of COPD has occurred or that some new lung disease has developed.

General health: *Have you gained or lost weight? Do you have joint pains? Do you eat nutritiously? Do you experience fevers, chills, or sweats?* A general inquiry such as this may disclose other health problems that can interfere with your ability to cope with COPD. Arthritis, for example, might complicate your ability to exercise for pulmonary rehabilitation.

Current lifestyle: *Do you feel that you've slowed down over the past few years? Do you get a good night's sleep? Do you exercise? Do you drink alcohol excessively? Do you take any medications?* A major part of COPD management is achieving and maintaining a healthy lifestyle and general level of fitness. Identifying any impediment to this can be critical.

The interview is also *your* opportunity to ask questions of your doctor. Don't pass it up. You need to put your two cents into the conversation. Some people may feel that asking questions will take up too much time or anger the doctor. But the doctor can't know what's on your mind and thus may not cover all the bases during the interview. If the doctor leaves any questions unanswered, make sure you speak up and ask! (Chapter 5 gives more suggestions on getting the most out of your visits to the doctor.)

The Physical Examination

Looking

Don't be surprised if your doctor gives you a good long stare during your appointment. In some cases, your appearance can reveal plenty about the general state of your health and, in particular, the condition of your lungs.

Here are some of the things your doctor will be looking for:

— **wider-than-normal chest.** Remember that emphysema sufferers have difficulty exhaling the air from their lungs. This results in lungs that are always overinflated, which can give the patient a barrel-chested appearance.
— **prominent neck muscles.** Breathing is hard work for someone with advanced COPD, and the normal breathing muscles — the diaphragm and the intercostal muscles located between the ribs —

HOW CAN YOU HELP PREPARE YOUR HEALTH HISTORY?
If you suspect you have COPD, or if you've been diagnosed with COPD and feel that your condition is changing, you can help your doctor by:

- **ensuring** the doctor has adequate information about you. If you're seeing a specialist for the first time, for example, phone ahead to ensure that the specialist has your file detailing your past treatments and results of lung function testing.
- **itemizing** your past lung and other health problems. Include details about your smoking history.
- **jotting** down facts so you don't forget the details. Accuracy is important. Maintain an ongoing diary of your symptoms and the drugs you're taking to keep track of important details concerning your COPD. *Don't* provide your doctor with an exhaustive list of every ailment you've ever suffered. *Do* provide a brief list of major health events, including hospitalizations, pneumonia, and lung infections, and details of any previous lung function testing (where, when, and the results).

can't do the job alone. So the neck muscles pitch in to help, and may appear to be straining with each breath.

— **weight.** People suffering predominantly from emphysema, especially if it's quite advanced, tend to be quite thin. Breathing is hard work for them and takes plenty of energy, keeping them on the lean side. Gaining weight and muscle mass can help here. Other people with COPD may be overweight, probably a result of the sedentary lifestyle their disease has imposed on them. Losing weight can help reduce breathlessness for these folks.

— **colour of lips, nails, and skin.** A blue or purple tone can indicate the possibility of cyanosis, a deficiency of oxygen in the blood.

— **breathing pattern.** Laboured breathing — for example, having to stop between sentences to catch a breath or breathing too fast — can be evidence of COPD or pulmonary fibrosis. Leaning forward to stabilize the chest for breathing can also be a sign of advanced COPD, usually emphysema.

— **swollen ankles.** Swollen ankles indicate edema, a condition where fluid collects in the tissues. In COPD patients, edema can be caused by the development of pulmonary hypertension due to low blood oxygen. Edema can also be a sign of congestive heart failure or of poor circulation to the legs.

Listening

Because COPD causes narrowing of the airways, the airflow through those tubes tends to be turbulent rather than streamlined. Just like water flowing in a turbulent brook, turbulent airflow makes noise. People with COPD are noisy breathers. Usually, it just seems that their breathing is louder than other people's, but sometimes you can hear whistling noises or wheezes even without a stethoscope.

Wheezing, which indicates an obstruction in your airways, may not be immediately apparent. At rest, many COPD patients aren't wheezy. Your doctor may be able to bring out wheezing by asking you to take a deep breath in and blow it out as forcefully and completely as possible. This forced exhalation will often reveal wheezes in COPD or asthma patients.

Your doctor may also count the time it takes you to blow out all the air you can. This test is called the **forced expiratory time** and is a simple form of lung function testing. Most people with healthy lungs can exhale completely in well under three seconds. An exhalation time over five seconds indicates abnormal airway obstruction. Some people with advanced COPD can take up to ten or twelve seconds to blow out all the air they can.

Listening for lung sounds with a stethoscope is called **auscultation**. By listening over the front, back, and sides of your chest while you breathe in and out, your doctor can cover all the major lobes of the lungs. In chronic bronchitis and asthma, the airways are swollen by inflammatory edema and secretions but not completely obstructed, making airflow very turbulent, so that wheezes tend to be quite noticeable.

However, the absence of wheezes does not rule out significant airway disease. In emphysema, for example, the airways tend to collapse shut during exhalation and airflow falls off dramatically, so that wheezes and even normal breath sounds may be absent — a sign of severe emphysematous airway obstruction. Other lung sounds, called **crackles**, are heard through the stethoscope mainly during inspiration. Crackles literally sound like "snap, crackle, pop," or the opening of a Velcro strap. These sounds come from the snapping open of tiny airways distorted shut by pulmonary fibrosis, or from a backup of fluid in the lungs (pulmonary edema) usually due to heart failure.

Touching

In a high-tech world, human touch seems hopelessly antiquated. But just as our eyes and ears can reveal volumes about the health of another, so can touch.

Percussion is one touch technique your doctor may use. Percussion, as its name indicates, involves lightly tapping the chest with the fingers. This makes the structures in the chest vibrate, and the quality of the sound produced can indicate the presence of disease. When the lungs are hyperinflated with air, as occurs with advanced COPD, the percussion note is very resonant — like striking an empty oil drum. When the lung is made more dense by disease like pneumonia, the percussion note becomes dull, as if the oil drum were filled. In other circumstances, the note is flat like tapping on your thigh muscle. This usually indicates a buildup of fluid around the lung in the pleural space — a **pleural effusion** — that can occur with infection, heart failure, or cancer.

Your doctor may also **palpate** ("touch gently" in Latin) your neck muscles, rib cage, and abdomen to reveal how well your breathing muscles are functioning. The doctor will be focusing on the function of your main breathing muscle — your diaphragm. A physical exam can often reveal whether your diaphragm has flattened out. Your diaphragm should be shaped like a dome, pointing upwards to your chest. When it pulls down, it brings air into your lungs. If it's permanently flattened, it can no longer do that effectively.

If the muscles of your neck are contracting to help with each breath, the doctor can feel this too. This is usually a sign that the lungs are hyper-inflated and that the diaphragm is flattened and weak, making help from these so-called accessory breathing muscles necessary.

Lung Function Testing

History taking and physical examination are essential elements of diagnosis, but often, especially in its early stages, COPD may not be strongly suggested by either process. In addition, not all smokers develop COPD, so there's often a subtle tendency by both smokers and doctors to overlook or deny the possibility of lung disease. That's what makes lung function testing so important. When done early in people in whom COPD is even remotely suggested or who are at risk for COPD, a simple test of lung function can reveal the hidden disease in its earliest stages better than any other diagnostic tool.

Edgar had a heart attack in 1980, nothing too serious. In fact, his doctor told him he could expect to be back to his normal activities in just a few months. He was only forty-five at the time. He was smoking heavily in those days — a pack or more each day. After the heart attack, he never did get his stamina back. Lots of activities went by the wayside. He had to give up his passion, martial arts. He felt winded all the time, exhausted. The doctors said it was just his heart and he should try to pace himself better. So he did. He slowed right down, giving up most of his physical activities. They made him too breathless anyway.

Today, Edgar is sixty-five and suffering from severe COPD. Based on his level of lung function, his respirologist has told him that he has only about a 60 percent chance of surviving for three years. Amazingly, Edgar's COPD was diagnosed only in 1995, and that diagnosis was a bit of a fluke. He was suffering one cold after another, so his family doctor sent him to an allergist for testing. After the testing revealed no allergies, the allergist asked him to blow into a small machine (a **spirometer**) to measure his lung function. That was the first time Edgar's lung function had ever been tested.

"I still remember what he said to me," recalls Edgar. "He said: 'Your lungs are shot. You've got emphysema.' Of course, hindsight is always 20/20, but I sure wish I'd had my lung function tested back in the early 1980s." Edgar figures that if he'd known back then that he was in the initial stages of COPD, he probably would have given up smoking and kept himself in better physical shape. Instead he smoked until 1990 and, worried about his heart condition, he lapsed into a fairly sedentary life. He figures that he wouldn't be in the condition he is now if his COPD had been diagnosed earlier.

Edgar's story has an important message: shortness of breath is a symptom that should never be overlooked, or underestimated, by the patient or doctor. We know that shortness of breath is a key sign of COPD, but it can also be associated with several other illnesses, such as heart failure or pulmonary fibrosis. Only through specific lung function testing can we properly evaluate the various potential causes of a person's breathlessness.

Lung function tests, or pulmonary function tests (PFTs), do exactly what their name says: they measure your breathing power. Your test results are measured against a set of normal, or predicted, standards. Comparing your results to these standard values helps your doctor determine your breathing capacity.

There are many ways to test lung function, but the tests most important for diagnosis of COPD are:

- **spirometry**, which provides a measure of airflow from the lungs ("spiro" is Greek for breathe),
- **diffusing capacity**, which determines how well gas is exchanged from the lungs to the blood,
- **oximetry** and **arterial blood gas analysis**, which measure how well the lungs are providing oxygen and removing carbon dioxide, and
- **exercise testing**, which can help identify the main reasons for shortness of breath.

Of these tests, spirometry is by far the best tool for early identification of COPD. It's also one of the simplest. It can often be performed in your doctor's office on a small machine. Diffusing capacity, blood gas analysis, and exercise testing must usually be performed in a PFT laboratory in a hospital or at a special clinic.

Spirometry

Spirometry is a simple procedure. First, clips are placed on your nose, so you will exhale only via your mouth. Next, you close your lips tightly around a small mouthpiece attached to the tubing of the spirometer and then you take a full breath in and hold it briefly. Then you are instructed to exhale into the spirometer as forcefully and as completely as you can for as long as you can. The spirometer measures the total amount of air you can blow out at one time and the speed of the airflow. If you can exhale plenty of air, that's great. A reduced amount of air could indicate a narrowing of the air passages in your lungs as occurs in COPD and asthma; a loss of lung tissue as occurs in emphysema; pulmonary fibrosis; or even a weakness of the chest and breathing muscles.

The spirometer itself can be a machine as large as a refrigerator or as small as a portable CD player. Spirometry testing is a team sport. To get an accurate reading requires maximum effort and concentration on your part. Don't be surprised when the person supervising the test starts shouting at you: "Keep blowing . . . keep blowing . . . Push! Push! Push!" You'll be quite red in the face by the end of the test if you've done a good job. Usually, you are asked to repeat the test three times, to ensure consistency.

During your spirometry test, you'll probably hear your doctor, nurse, or respiratory therapist talk about measuring your FEV_1 (pronounced F-E-V-one), FVC, and the FEV_1/FVC ratio. You might hear them talk about how your measurements are a certain percentage of predicted values. A small computer in the spirometer will probably print out a graph with these terms and a lot of numbers. It's easy to get lost in the technical jargon, but actually, the terms are pretty self-explanatory.

Figure 4.1 on the next page explains what is being measured by the spirometry test.

There are predicted values for a person's FEV_1. We know what the normal, or predicted, value should be for a person of a certain age, height, sex, and ethnic background. For example, the predicted FEV_1 for a sixty-five-year-old Caucasian woman of average height and weight without COPD might be in the range of 2.5 L. If that woman has COPD, she can't blow air out of her obstructed airways easily, and her FEV_1 will be less than the predicted values for her age, height, sex, and ethnic background. How much less helps to determine the severity of her COPD.

FIGURE 4.1: THE SPIROMETRY TEST

Term	What It Means
FVC Forced vital capacity (measured in litres)	You're asked to inhale deeply and exhale as much air as possible. The total amount of air exhaled — **forced** out — is called the **vital capacity.**
FEV_1 Forced expiratory volume in one second (measured litres)	This is the amount of air you exhale in the first one second of breathing in out forcefully.
FEV_1**/FVC ratio**	This is the relationship between the amount of air you can exhale in one second and the total amount of air you can exhale completely. This tells you the proportion of the vital capacity you can exhale in one second of blowing.

In a way, FEV_1 tells us how "old" your lungs are. As we age, so do our lungs. The FEV_1 for a healthy sixty-year-old is less than that for a healthy twenty-year-old. The average rate of decline of FEV_1 with age is about 15 to 20 mL per year, which is not very much, actually. If you smoke cigarettes and are susceptible to the effects of cigarettes, your age-related decline in FEV_1 will be greater — up to 80 mL per year in some cases.

The lungs of a person suffering from COPD function as if they were older than those of someone who does not have COPD. A COPD patient's FEV_1 can tell us a lot about his or her prognosis, symptoms, tolerance for exercise, and even expected lifespan. Everyone with lung disease should know their FEV_1, and so should their doctors. It's like knowing your blood pressure if you have hypertension or your blood sugar if you have diabetes. FEV_1 is just as important for those with COPD.

Here are the general rules for someone with COPD:

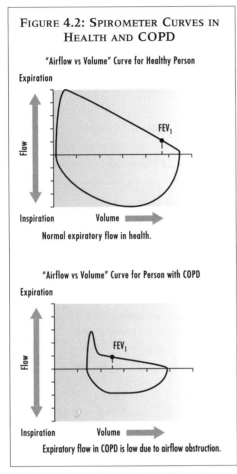

FIGURE 4.2: SPIROMETER CURVES IN HEALTH AND COPD

"Airflow vs Volume" Curve for Healthy Person

Expiration

Flow

FEV_1

Inspiration   Volume

Normal expiratory flow in health.

"Airflow vs Volume" Curve for Person with COPD

Expiration

Flow

FEV_1

Inspiration   Volume

Expiratory flow in COPD is low due to airflow obstruction.

— If FEV_1 is 70 percent of the predicted value, you're suffering from **mild** COPD.

— If it is 50 to 69 percent of the predicted value, you are suffering from **moderate** COPD.

— If it is less than 50 percent of the predicted value, you're suffering from **severe** COPD.

Like all rules, there are exceptions. The terms "mild," "moderate," and "severe" are qualitative terms used as a guide to estimating the severity or impact of COPD. FEV_1 doesn't tell the whole story about COPD severity, however. For example, there is only a general relationship between a patient's FEV_1 and the degree of breathlessness experienced from COPD. It's not uncommon for one COPD patient with a certain FEV_1 to complain of extreme breathlessness, while another COPD sufferer with the same FEV_1 experiences only mild to moderate breathlessness. This is partly because the sensation of breathlessness is influenced by many factors in addition to the level of lung function or FEV_1. Such factors include the patient's general level of fitness, weight, muscle strength, heart function, personality, and tolerance for pain and breathlessness.

Arthur is a good example of someone with advanced COPD (his FEV_1 is only 21 percent of predicted value) who is nevertheless able to function at a relatively high level because he is highly motivated and able to work at keeping himself in the best possible shape by exercising regularly.

Because FEV_1 doesn't always predict a given person's performance or comfort level in COPD, doctors are beginning to try to measure what is called "health status" or "quality of life" as a guide to managing the symptoms of people with COPD. Health status measurements usually involve answering a questionnaire dealing with such things as breathlessness, physical function, emotional function, and the ability to cope with COPD.

The FVC, or forced vital capacity, is also measured during spirometry. Normally, about 70 to 80 percent of the vital capacity is exhaled during the first one second. That means the FEV_1/FVC ratio is about 0.70 to 0.80. In COPD, however, FEV_1 is low because of airway obstruction, so the FEV_1/FVC ratio tends to be low too (less than 0.70). Early on,

---

DO YOU KNOW YOUR FEV_1?

You should! If you don't, it's a simple thing to find out. If you smoke, and if you know you have COPD or even suspect it, ask your doctor to arrange for a spirometry test. When you have the test, ask the respiratory therapist or doctor for an explanation of the readings. Focus on your FEV_1. If you are not told what it is, make sure you ask! It's measured in litres, and you should ask how your FEV_1 compares to predicted values for persons of normal health. That will give you an idea of how severe your COPD is.

In an effort to help smokers quit, some doctors calculate the "FEV_1 age," or "lung age," for their patients. Here's an example. A fifty-year-old smoker complains to his family doctor that he is more breathless than last year when walking up hills on the golf course. He's also noticed a slight cough most days that produces a little white phlegm. He calls it his smoker's cough. Since he is a long-time smoker his doctor astutely suspects early COPD and orders a spirometry test. For our 170-cm-tall smoking golfer, the predicted FEV_1 is 3.58 L — but his measured FEV_1 is 3.0 L. Doesn't seem too bad. But when his doctor calculated his lung age, our fifty-year-old golfer learned that he had the lungs of a seventy-five-year-old! (The predicted FEV_1 of a healthy seventy-five-year-old man is approximately 3.0 L.)

What's your FEV_1? Are you still smoking? Knowing your FEV_1 can also be helpful if you ever end up in an emergency department because of your COPD. The doctors treating you may not have access to your medical records and this information can help them treat you better.

Here's how you can calculate the predicted values for FEV_1 (in litres) for a person of your age (in years) and height (in centimetres):

Women: $FEV_1 = (0.0414 \times height) - (0.0244 \times age) - 2.190$
Men: $FEV_1 = (0.0342 \times height) - (0.0255 \times age) - 1.578$

If you know what your measured FEV_1 is and you don't mind a little more arithmetic, you can figure out what your "lung age" is. Simply insert your measured FEV_1 (in litres) and your height (in centimetres) into the appropriate equation above, and solve for age.

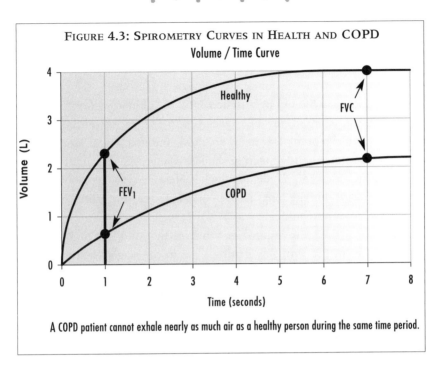

FIGURE 4.3: SPIROMETRY CURVES IN HEALTH AND COPD
Volume / Time Curve

A COPD patient cannot exhale nearly as much air as a healthy person during the same time period.

when COPD is mild, FVC remains in the normal range and only FEV_1 or FEV_1/FVC are reduced. As the disease progresses, eventually both FEV_1 and FVC will be lower than normal, but the FEV_1/FVC ratio will always be reduced.

Let's look at another real example. Janet is sixty-five. On her first visit to the respirologist in 1997, her FEV_1 was 0.72 L, or 33 percent of the predicted value for a woman her age. Her FVC was 1.75 L, 61 percent predicted. Her FEV_1/FVC ratio was 0.41, also relatively low. That meant she was suffering from severe COPD.

"I had my first spirometry test back in 1992," Janet says. "My family doctor suspected I had COPD and he sent me to the hospital for the test. Sure enough, he made the diagnosis based on my results. I never thought to ask what the results of the test meant. It wasn't until I was in a reha-bilitation program in 1998 that I realized that I should be paying attention to my results because they could tell me a lot about the progress of my COPD — whether my condition was stabilized or getting worse. But I still didn't ask to be told the details. For example, at that time, I couldn't tell you what FEV_1 meant. It wasn't until I was in a study for a new COPD medication that I began to understand the graphs and the measurements. All I did was ask the respiratory therapist to explain things to me. It was my own fault for not learning this earlier. It was just a matter of asking a simple question.

"Now I know what my FEV_1 is and I follow it along with my doctors. When I was last tested, my FEV_1 was 0.83 L, or 38 percent predicted. That sounds like a pretty low mark on a test, and it is. But at least I know that it hasn't deteriorated much in the last few years, and that's reassuring. In fact, my FEV_1 is slightly higher than it was in 1997, which probably means that my lungs have been able to respond a little bit to the medications I'm now taking.

"Because I asked, my respirologist told me that an FEV_1 of 38 percent predicted means I'm probably getting close to the stage when my blood carbon dioxide level will start to rise. By itself, that's not dangerous, but it is a sign that I'm slowly running out of lung power. Again, because I asked, he told me that, statistically speaking at least, this level of lung function means that I have about a 25 percent chance of dying from my COPD in the next three years. That's a sobering thought, but it's something I feel I need to know."

Post-Bronchodilator Spirometry
Although spirometry testing can't distinguish between emphysema and chronic bronchitis, it can often reveal whether a patient is also suffering from asthma or a combination of COPD and asthma. One of the things that distinguishes COPD from asthma is the presence or absence of reversible airflow obstruction — that is, obstruction that lessens in response to bronchodilator medications. In common parlance, the FEV_1 is said to "reverse" or "revert" to normal.

To make the distinction, the patient will be tested before and after inhaling bronchodilator medication. In asthmatic patients, this medication relaxes the muscles around the airways, opening up the bronchial tubes, making breathing easier by increasing the amount of air that can be exhaled, thus increasing the measured FEV_1 (a 15 to 20 percent improvement is considered a positive test). COPD patients, on the other hand, usually demonstrate only a slight improvement in response to bronchodilator medication (5 to 10 percent). FEV_1 doesn't tell the whole story, however, since some COPD patients seem to function much better when taking bronchodilators, even though their FEV_1 values don't change much during the bronchodilator test. This suggests that for some people the bronchodilators are helping by changing some other aspects of lung function that are not measured by FEV_1. It could be that for these people, bronchodilators are helping to reduce the amount of lung hyperinflation, which could lead to less breathlessness.

In other cases, FEV_1 will improve only when larger than conventional doses of bronchodilator are taken or if more than one type of bronchodilator (e.g., salbutamol plus ipratropium) are taken at the same time. The respirologist is often the best person to help sort out these unusual responses.

Diffusing Capacity

Oxygen is breathed into the body, carbon dioxide is exhaled. Those gases are exchanged in the lungs through a process called **diffusion**. Measuring the diffusing capacity gives us a good idea of how efficiently the lungs are exchanging gas from the lung to the blood. Specifically, this test focuses on how well the delicate alveoli are working. The diffusing capacity test involves breathing in a mixture of gas containing a tiny and safe amount of carbon monoxide and then holding your breath for a few seconds. When you exhale, the exhaled air is analyzed for the amount of carbon monoxide remaining. The difference between what goes in and what comes out tells us how much of the carbon monoxide has diffused from the lungs into the blood. This gives us a measure of how much of the lung's huge surface area is healthy and available for efficient gas exchange.

For someone with emphysema, the diffusing capacity will be lower than that predicted for a healthy person, because the emphysema results in alveolar and airway destruction, so there is less lung tissue available for gas exchange. The diffusing capacity is very sensitive and is often abnormally low before the FEV_1 starts to fall. A low diffusion capacity may, therefore, be the earliest sign that emphysema is present. The diffusing capacity can be measured only in a sophisticated PFT laboratory.

Oximetry and Arterial Blood Gas Analysis

Like diffusing capacity testing, these tests measure the efficiency of oxygenation and of carbon dioxide removal by the lungs. Oximetry, often available in the doctor's office, is a simple, painless method of measuring the degree to which your hemoglobin is saturated with oxygen. Hemoglobin, a component of blood, is the main molecule responsible for transporting oxygen throughout the body and is normally saturated with oxygen to a value of 92 to 98 percent. The symbol for oxyhemoglobin saturation is SO_2%. The lower the SO_2%, the lower the saturation of oxygen in the blood. Measurement of SO_2% is called **oximetry**. The oximeter is a simple infrared probe that is clipped to the finger or earlobe. The oximeter records the colour of light reflected from your blood. The redder the blood, the higher the oxygen content.

Arterial blood gas analysis is a more invasive procedure, requiring that blood be taken with a needle inserted into an artery, usually at the wrist. This test measures oxyhemoglobin saturation (SO_2%), together with the pressure of oxygen (PO_2) and carbon dioxide in the blood (PCO_2). Both PO_2 and PCO_2 are measured in millimetres of mercury, abbreviated as mmHg. The test also measures the acidity of the blood — its pH. (See Figure 4.4.) In advanced COPD, the PO_2 and SO_2% are often low. This condition is called **hypoxemia**. The PCO_2, however, is often higher than normal, indicating that the lungs are having trouble getting rid of the waste gas, carbon dioxide. This condition is called **hypercarbia** and it leads to **respiratory acidosis** in which the arterial pH is lower than normal.

FIGURE 4.4: NORMAL RANGES AND CRITICAL LEVELS

Test	Normal Ranges	Critical Levels
SO_2%	92–98%	less than 85–88%
PO_2	95–98 mmHg	less than 55 mmHg
PCO_2	37–43 mmHg	more than 50 mmHg
pH	7.37–7.43	less than 7.30

When the SO_2% or PO_2 remain below the so-called critical levels, lung disease is usually extensive and supplemental oxygen therapy in the home may be necessary. Chapter 11 discusses home oxygen.

Exercise Testing
Exercise testing is usually used when the cause of breathlessness is not clear. By exercising the heart, lungs, and muscles, the contributions of

each can be separately analyzed. Using a stationary bicycle or a treadmill, you will be asked to exercise in a controlled fashion until you are breathless. While exercising, your blood pressure, oxygen levels, breathing rate, and ventilation (the amount of air breathed in and out) are monitored. In addition, your heart activity is monitored by an electrocardiogram (ECG).

We know with some precision how the body responds to exercise. We expect, for example, the heart rate and ventilation to increase above resting values as exercise progresses. Exercise testing can be very helpful in sorting out the main cause of breathlessness when other testing has been inconclusive. For example, if breathlessness is mainly due to heart disease, the heart rate response to exercise is exaggerated, while the breathing rate or ventilation tends to stay in the normal range. If lung disease is the main culprit, patients usually stop exercising because they have reached their maximum breathing rates and maximum ventilation, while the heart response to exercise follows a normal pattern. Low levels of blood oxygenation, not detectable at rest, can also be uncovered by measuring $SO_2\%$ continuously during exercise. Exercise testing can also reveal when poor physical condition, as opposed to heart or lung disease, is the main cause of breathlessness with exertion.

Other Tests

Chest X-rays: Although a chest X-ray alone won't provide a definitive diagnosis of COPD, it can suggest the presence of lung hyperinflation as a sign of advanced COPD (see Figure 2.2). The chest X-ray can also be very helpful in ruling out other health problems such as lung cancer, pulmonary fibrosis, heart problems, and infections, including pneumonia. A specialized computerized scan of the lungs called a **CT (computed tomography) scan** is often used to show greater detail in the lungs. It is especially useful in documenting the degree of emphysema, in diagnosing pulmonary fibrosis and bronchiectasis, and in determining the extent of cancer.

Figure 4.5 is a CT scan of a patient with COPD and advanced emphysema, mainly on one lung. The "Swiss cheese" effect from the lung holes is obvious.

Allergy Testing: Occasionally, allergic reactions to common allergens like pollens, dusts, and animal dander can induce an asthmatic-like bronchoconstriction reaction in people with COPD, which will only worsen the breathlessness already present. These reactions are usually self-evident, but if you suspect that allergies may be interfering with your COPD management ask your doctor to refer you for allergy testing. This usually consists of an allergist injecting a series of common

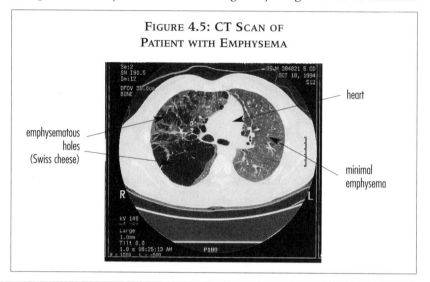

FIGURE 4.5: CT SCAN OF
PATIENT WITH EMPHYSEMA

heart

emphysematous
holes
(Swiss cheese)

minimal
emphysema

R

L

"YOU HAVE COPD" — DEALING WITH THE NEWS OF DIAGNOSIS

Dealing with the initial diagnosis of COPD is tough. First of all, you're being told that you're not a perfect specimen. You are "diseased." You may not feel all that well, you might deny your symptoms, and you may even be angry. Reactions are as diverse as the people suffering from COPD. Arthur's wife, a nurse, suspected Arthur had COPD long before he was actually diagnosed. Arthur, on the other hand, lived in denial, hoping that his lungs would return to normal once he quit smoking. It took him many years to come to terms with the disease. For Janet, the diagnosis of COPD was, in a way, good news. She'd convinced herself that the lung problems she was experiencing were a sign of cancer. Louise felt beaten by her diagnosis of COPD. Because her career was finished, she felt that her life was at an end.

The second problem you face when confronted with a diagnosis is fear. "Does this mean I'm going to die prematurely?" "Will I suffer?" These feelings are natural and they need to be dealt with in a constructive way.

Like your physical symptoms, your feelings about your disease deserve attention. As Janet says: "COPD is a disease of the head *and* the lungs. Not being able to breathe properly can throw your head into a real tizzy." Knowledge is everything. Knowing about your disease and how it can respond to treatment will help give you the strength to cope with it. That's why working with your doctor and other health professionals to regularly update your knowledge about the state of your COPD — and your emotions — is so important to staying well. See chapter 6 for more about the emotional elements of COPD.

allergens just under your skin and watching for mild swelling and inflammation, indicating an allergic reaction. If allergies are confirmed, your allergist will give you detailed advice on how to avoid contact with the specific allergens and how to control your symptoms. If the allergist prescribes any medications, be sure to verify with your family doctor that these new drugs are compatible with any other medications you are taking.

Airway Challenge Test: If you are prone to sudden bouts of rapid-onset breathlessness when exposed to strong smells, cold air, or certain dusts, you may have an element of asthma ("twitchy airways") complicating your COPD. If you or your doctor suspect that you might have a significant component of asthma, the first test should be to determine whether your FEV_1 will improve by more than 20 percent in response to an inhaled bronchodilator such as salbutamol. If so, this medication should be part of your COPD management plan and your doctor may also want to consider adding an inhaled corticosteroid. (Chapter 10 provides more details on medications.)

If the FEV_1 test with salbutamol is negative, but asthma is still suspected, an airway challenge test may be done. This test attempts to provoke a "hidden" asthma component. The test consists of two parts: breathing in increasing concentrations of a mist containing methacholine or histamine (two chemicals that can provoke asthmatic bronchoconstriction in people with a tendency to asthma) and repeated measuring of FEV_1. Once again, if the test reveals that a component of asthma is pres-ent, then your COPD therapy should be augmented with anti-asthma medications.

5

COPD as a Team Sport — Working Together with Your Doctor

We handed this chapter to Arthur to write for us. He tells us, in his words, about working with his doctor (and other health professionals) and getting the most out of their relationship. We couldn't have said it better.

*I*n my younger, healthier days, I loved sports and played on many baseball and softball teams. I learned that a team, working together, can accomplish much more than an individual working on his own. That's how I approach COPD — it's a team effort. Together with the help of my team, I feel I've stabilized the progress of my COPD and that I'm "in control." My lungs may not be getting any better, but, more important, I'm not getting any worse. I learned a long time ago that I'm going to have to live with this thing.

So, who's on my COPD team? My wife, Bev, is a key player, together with my family doctor, our pharmacists (they're husband and wife), and my respiratory therapist. Quarterbacking the team is my respirologist.

I visit my respirologist at least once each year, unless I have a flare-up. In those cases, I contact his secretary immediately. I've been seeing the same respirologist for over ten years, so we have a good routine worked out now. He's a plain-talking fellow. I know that's not everybody's preference but that's the kind of care I like. The two of us can have a frank

DO I NEED A FAMILY DOCTOR?

The short answer is *yes!* Anyone with a chronic illness like COPD should have a family physician, the professional who knows your complete medical history.

Although your respirologist or internist may be the quarterback for your COPD, your family doctor is the team owner, whose job it is to coordinate all the other players while staying focused on the bottom line: your continued good health.

It is very inefficient and basically wrong to manage your health and diseases solely by relying on a few specialists acting independently without a family doctor to tie them all together and consider the whole person — you!

DO I NEED A RESPIROLOGIST?

Your family physician has told you that you have COPD. You're feeling pretty good; the drugs your family doctor prescribed seem to be working well for you. But you're wondering whether you need to see a specialist. If you're concerned, ask your family doctor whether you need to be referred to a respirologist, a specialist in diagnosing and treating disorders of the respiratory system, specifically the lungs.

Most people with COPD do not need to see a respirologist. They can develop and manage a preventative maintenance program in cooperation with their family physicians. Remember that a respirologist attends only to the condition of your lungs. Your family doctor tends to your overall health care. Your respirologist and your family doctor should be communicating about your condition. Be on the safe side, however, and always ask each whether he or she has communicated with the other about your condition.

A referral to a respirologist may be a good idea if

- your COPD is very advanced, based on initial lung function testing
- you remain very breathless despite initial attempts at drug therapy
- your diagnosis is in question (your family doctor is not certain whether you have COPD or some other disorder)
- you are confused about your diagnosis (you're not sure whether you have COPD or asthma, for example)
- you've been hospitalized with an ailment related to your COPD — a lung infection, for example
- you're suffering from frequent flare-ups of your COPD
- you cough up blood or develop persistent chest pain
- your chest X-ray shows something suspicious that suggests cancer (even if you are feeling relatively well)
- your ankles begin to swell
- you or your family doctor is wondering whether you would benefit from oxygen therapy
- you have been started on oxygen therapy

discussion. He tells me exactly where I stand and what I can expect in the future. I like to hear all the news, both good and bad.

He's always been clear about the severity of my condition. My level of lung function is quite low. Looking at both my level of lung function — as measured by the FEV_1 in the lab (about 21 percent of the predicted normal value) — and my degree of breathlessness, my COPD is in the advanced stages, although not so far advanced that I need supplemental oxygen in the house. Despite this, I've been able to remain physically active. My doctor has always encouraged me to stay busy, assuring me it's safe as long as I pace myself. He finds it amazing that I can accomplish as much as I do. Most people with my level of lung function can't (or won't) be as active as I am. That's a good message for me. I like to know I'm doing as well as I possibly can and I want to know the precise details of my condition. The encouragement is good too.

If I wasn't happy with the treatment I was receiving, I would definitely switch doctors or, at the very least, ask for a second opinion.

Planning for the Visit

Each year, about the same time, I call my respirologist's secretary and book an appointment. It makes sense to keep on top of my COPD. I want to keep my condition as stable as possible since COPD is something I've got to live with for the rest of my life. That means getting together and

JANET'S STORY

In Janet's case, her family doctor advised her to see a respirologist four years after he diagnosed her COPD. Janet initially started on salbutamol, and things went pretty well until 1996, when she experienced a string of lung infections she couldn't shake. "At that point, my family doctor decided it was time for me to see a respirologist, and I agreed," recalls Janet.

After a battery of testing (including chest X-rays and spirometry), her respirologist confirmed the diagnosis of emphysema and changed her medications radically. In addition, Janet attended a twelve-week pulmonary rehabilitation program on her respirologist's recommendation. Going to a respirologist has brought Janet peace of mind. "For me, COPD is as much a disease of the head as of the lungs," she explains. For Janet, anxiety equals breathlessness. Seeing a respirologist has alleviated many of her anxieties, allowing her to feel more in control of her breathlessness. "I feel I now know more about COPD and the specifics of my condition. I feel reassured by that." And knowing that she can call on the services of an expert whenever she needs them gives Janet that extra level of confidence she requires to feel comfortable with her COPD.

talking about the preventative maintenance plan that my respirologist, my family doctor, and I have developed over the years. This plan includes the drugs I take, plus the work I do myself to stay healthy — like walking, getting annual flu shots, and keeping my weight in check. I figure it makes sense to visit my doctor when I'm feeling good. That way, I can make sure to keep doing the right things.

I know the doctor is a busy guy, so I always call about six to eight weeks before I want to see him. Specialists sometimes have to book non-urgent appointments months in advance, so I make sure I don't leave things to the last minute. I've made certain to meet and talk with his secretary when I've been in for previous appointments, so she knows who she's talking to when I phone. It always helps when people know who you are. That way, if I'm concerned about something, and would like an early or extra appointment, I always feel like I'm on the inside track.

Bev doesn't come with me to every visit, but I like it when she does. I'm really lucky because my wife is the director of nursing at our local hospital. She knows a lot about my condition, so she can be a big help when I'm talking with the doctor. Also it helps to have another set of ears at the appointment. Bev is my backup. A lot of what we talk about is pretty technical and we discuss many different topics. It's great that Bev

WHAT CAN I EXPECT FROM A RESPIROLOGIST?

A respirologist will often do one or more of the following:

- make an in-depth assessment of your diagnosis and symptoms (expect to be examined and tested by the respirologist)
- perform an airway challenge test to diagnose hidden asthma, if necessary
- make medication adjustments, if necessary
- check your inhaler technique
- assess the need for home oxygen therapy
- arrange for a bronchoscopy test, if needed
- assess the need for and coordinate a pulmonary rehabilitation program, if required
- refer you to a heart specialist, if required (e.g., for breathlessness out of keeping with the measured lung function)
- provide your family doctor with information about your condition and the medications prescribed
- coordinate a preventative maintenance program with you and your family doctor, including devising an action plan to deal with COPD flare-ups
- answer all your questions regarding your COPD

and I can compare notes at the end of an appointment. If I do get into trouble with my COPD and end up hospitalized, I want Bev to be comfortable dealing with my doctor, and I want him to know her. Bev has my power of attorney for personal care. That means that if for some reason I can't make my own decisions about my health care, Bev has the legal power to act on my behalf. So I want her to be just as knowledgeable about my condition as I am. Coming to my appointments with me gives her the information she needs.

My visits to the respirologist are all-day affairs. Because we live far from the hospital I don't plan anything else for the day. I don't want to feel rushed and I don't want to get myself into a panic that could result in breathing difficulties.

I prepare for the day like I prepare for any big event in my life now. Any day that's different from my normal routine can cause extra breathlessness, and I don't want that to happen. I know I'm already a bit concerned about the drive into Ottawa and anxious about getting a parking spot close enough to the hospital. So I start out by being organized, keeping everything under control.

I start by getting ready ahead of time. The night before, I set out my clothes and other things I need to take with me so that I won't be in a rush before I leave the house. I make sure to bring along all the medications I'm using, and I prepare a list of what I want to talk to the doctor about. All of this preparation means that I can sit back and relax for a few minutes before leaving the house.

My respirologist's office is in the Ottawa Hospital, a building that covers at least two city blocks. Some of the parking is hundreds of metres away from the entrance. Even though I have a handicapped parking permit, the handicapped spots are often filled. In the winter (I find it very difficult to catch my breath in cold weather), I need to be let off at the front door of the hospital, so I can get inside and let my lungs warm up. That's when Bev drives me. She'll drop me off and then park the car. In the warmer months, I drive myself, arriving at the hospital early enough to find a place close to where I'm going.

I've learned to ask for help if I need it at the hospital. I don't try to tough it out. One day, I had an appointment with both my orthopedic surgeon (I have an artificial hip) and my respirologist. I also needed to have a chest X-ray. Three different places to go in the same hospital, but all at different corners of the building. First, I thought very carefully about where to park my car and I walked very slowly to my first appointment, stopping a couple of times along the way. After that appointment, I requested a wheelchair to get to my next two appointments. That way, I was able to get everything done without becoming too breathless.

Here's another thing I've learned in my years with COPD — be honest.

GOAL SETTING WITH YOUR COPD TEAM

It's one thing to treat flare-ups of your COPD; it's quite another to develop a long-term vision of how you want the next weeks, months, and years of your life with COPD to unfold. You and your family doctor (and your respirologist, if you have one) should talk together about the long-term goals you want to set for yourself and your COPD.

Four general topics warrant discussion:

- prevention of further damage to your lungs,
- relief of symptoms and optimization of your general fitness, nutrition, mental outlook, and coping skills,
- an action plan to deal with flare-ups, and
- a plan for eventual end-of-life decision making, when appropriate (see "Tough Choices, Difficult Decisions" in chapter 14)

Some of the specifics you'll want to talk about with your doctor include

- tackling smoking cessation, if you haven't already quit
- establishing an early diagnosis of COPD and keeping current on any changes in your condition
- identifying whether your disease has an asthmatic component
- documenting and following the level of activity that causes breathlessness (that is, figuring out what this means for everyday living)
- finding ways to be as physically fit and well nourished as possible
- learning about ways to prevent recurrent flare-ups of your COPD
- treating flare-ups promptly and effectively to minimize symptoms (developing your action plan)
- identifying any other diseases you may have (e.g., heart problems) that can affect your COPD
- discussing your fears and the ways you cope with your COPD at home, socially, and at work
- talking about the impact of your disease on your family life and the possible future ramifications of the disease for your caregivers
- discovering procedures to help you cope better or more effectively
- discussing the possibilities of future drug treatment or the possibility of oxygen therapy
- discussing your wishes for end-of-life decisions

You should be talking about all aspects of your life, some of which — your sex life, for example — you may consider extremely private. That means one thing: you need to have a doctor whom you feel comfortable talking to and who is comfortable helping you deal with these personal issues.

When I go to the doctor, I am totally upfront about my condition. I don't try to sugarcoat. I used to be very proud. I'd try to make the best of things and downplay how lousy I was feeling. That is not the way to get the best care. Your doctor needs to know the precise details about you and your health. Otherwise, how can he or she give you the best help? I learned this lesson from watching my father go to the doctor. My dad — he died in 1999 — had emphysema too.

Dad was a farmer and he was often breathless when working. When he visited the doctor, however, he'd be put into a wheelchair and pushed into the clinic. Since he hadn't exerted himself, Dad's oxygen levels would be fine and he wouldn't appear breathless at all. The doctor didn't question Dad about the extent of his condition (as he should have), nor did Dad reveal any information about his breathlessness (as he should have). As a result, I don't think Dad got the best treatment for his emphysema. In this case, the team wasn't working well together.

A lot of this is pride. It's hard to tell the doctor you're not as healthy as you once were or not as healthy as you want to be. It took me a long time to be able to convince *myself* that there were things I could no longer do. But I've come to the realization that to get the best treatment possible, I must be as honest as I can about how I am and how I feel. The doctor needs to have the straight goods. And I try to give him that information — warts and all. In return, I expect the same from the doctor.

Using a Checklist

This year's appointment with my respirologist was pretty ordinary. It was in the winter, so Bev and I went in together. I was prepared with my usual checklist. I wanted to

- review all the drugs (prescribed by all my doctors) I'm currently using,
- ask for any new drugs that might be helpful to me, and
- review the results of my breathing test to determine where I stand relative to my last appointment.

I had a couple of extra items on my list. Bev and I would soon be taking a Caribbean cruise, and I wanted to know whether any precautions should be taken, anything I should be concerned about. Also, I'm finding breathing increasingly difficult in the cold weather. I wanted to know if that meant my COPD was getting worse. If I have a question, I ask it. No question is a dumb one, I've learned.

The Visit

My appointment started with a breathing test. The respiratory therapist is usually the same person, and by now we know each other quite well. We always start each breathing test with the same exchange. She asks me how I'm doing and I reply: "Well, I'm still here!" I've always found that a kind

---

WHAT SHOULD I BRING TO MY FIRST APPOINTMENT WITH A RESPIROLOGIST?

- *All* of the medications you are currently taking for COPD and any other conditions (even non-pulmonary conditions; and don't forget inhalers — they're drugs too). Drug interactions can have negative side effects. There can be too many cooks (doctors) stirring the pot — and adding and changing the ingredients (drugs) along the way. It's in your own best interest to keep all the cooks informed of all the drugs you're taking. This includes any natural, herbal, or alternative medications you are using. These remedies may be very potent and can interact with your prescription drugs.
- **A brief synopsis of your lung health history.** When did you start smoking? When did you stop? If you haven't stopped, when are you planning to stop? Do you want help quitting? If your attempts to quit have been unsuccessful, what made them fail? Have you ever been exposed to any unusual pollutants, including fumes, dusts, or vapours? Does anyone else in your family have COPD?
- **The details of your COPD.** A diary is helpful in these instances. It can be a simple journal of point-form entries detailing when you started noticing breathing difficulties, what triggers your breathlessness, dates of hospitalizations, dates of lung infections, and drugs you've been prescribed over the years and your reactions to them.
- **A short general health history.** Do you have any allergies? Any other chronic illnesses?
- **Another person.** You'll be hearing lots of detailed information. Another person can help you remember everything that was said during the appointment.
- **A list of questions you want answered about your COPD.** To make certain that you've covered everything, begin making the list well in advance of your appointment.
- **A "don't take anything for granted" attitude.** If the explanations given to you aren't clear, or if you are confused about something, ask again!

Like Arthur, remember to check your pride at the door. You won't get the best treatment unless you're honest with yourself and your doctor about the nature and extent of your COPD symptoms.

---

word together with a smile — and remembering to say "please" and "thank you" — goes a long way.

My respiratory therapist is great. The spirometry test yields the best results only if you put out your maximum effort. To make me produce my best effort, she really gets into it, cheering me on to exhale as much as I possibly can. By the end of the process, she's as red in the face as I am. I pay attention to the results. Over the years, I've learned what the different values are. This year, I was happy with my FEV_1. I was in great form and it was actually a little better than last year's result.

I headed back to the respirologist's office, spirometry results in hand. Here's a quick list of some of the topics we covered in this year's appointment:

— my **spirometry results**
— whether I need to be using **supplemental oxygen**
— **drugs** I'm currently taking, how I'm taking them (especially my inhaler technique), and whether they're effective or whether I could or should stop taking them
— whether I can or should change the **doses** of any of these drugs as needed (in the case of a flare-up, for example)
— **new drugs** I might consider taking
— my **sleeping patterns**, especially breathlessness at night
— episodes of **unusual breathlessness** and their causes
— whether my ankles are **swelling** or my fingertips are turning blue
— whether I was **coughing** or producing phlegm
— whether I had spit **blood**, seen blood in phlegm, or had **chest pain**
— the **flu vaccine** and new medications for treatment of the flu
— maintaining a **healthy weight** and a healthy diet
— staying in the best **physical shape**
— the possibility of attending a **rehabilitation program**
— my current **activities** (both work and pleasure)
— ways to deal with the **cold weather**
— a review of my **action plan** for a flare-up of my COPD
— **travelling**, in particular flying
— an **overall review of my health** (How do I feel I'm doing? Am I still enjoying life?)

Reviewing the Details

I'll give you a few of the details. On this visit my respirologist had arranged that I be given extra doses of Combivent — a mixture of two different types of bronchodilators combined in a single puffer — during the lung function tests. He wanted to see whether the combination would be of any benefit for me, and how much, if any, my FEV_1 could improve if we decided to try a higher dosage.

Also, since I was using six to eight puffs of salbutamol on most days, he gave me a sample of a longer-acting bronchodilator called formoterol in the Turbuhaler format (Oxeze) to try, partly because he wanted to see whether I preferred the Turbuhaler dry powder inhaler to another puffer. I'm always willing to try something new. I'll report back to the respirologist immediately if it doesn't work, or if I experience any unwanted or odd side effects.

Getting your drug regimen right is important. Here's a little story about drugs. I'm always glad to have Bev along when we talk about drugs. All of the many details surrounding each drug can get quite confusing — how you take it, when you take it, the dosage you should be taking. In fact, I

ARTHUR'S ACTION PLAN FOR A COPD FLARE-UP

This is the action plan my respirologist and I have put together in the event that my COPD flares up. A "flare-up" means a progressive worsening over a few days of breathlessness and fatigue without an obvious cause. It will often be accompanied by a fever and a new or worsening cough and more phlegm, yellow or green in colour, that may be harder than normal to raise from my lungs.

Here's my step-by-step plan:

- Try to relieve breathlessness by taking extra doses of my bronchodilator (up to two to four puffs every couple of hours, if necessary).
- Rest. Don't overdo it.
- Drink plenty of fluids and take acetaminophen for aches and pains.
- If there is worsening or no improvement after one or two days and especially if there is more cough and phlegm, start taking antibiotic and cortisone tablets as directed. Phone the doctor.
- If at any time during the flare-up I get worse, phone the doctor or go to the emergency department.

This is *my* plan. If you suffer from COPD, you should speak to your doctor about developing your own plan. For example, not all COPD flare-ups require an antibiotic or cortisone. But because of my advanced COPD, my doctor and I have decided that I should take both early on during a flare-up. (COPD flare-ups are discussed in greater depth in Chapter 14.)

did get confused once. When I started taking an inhaled corticosteroid I used it only when I felt I needed it. I didn't understand that I needed to take it twice daily on a regular basis. My pharmacist called me on it. Because I wasn't coming into the pharmacy for a repeat prescription, he could tell that I wasn't using it as prescribed. That taught me two important lessons. First, it's great to have a team working with you, and my pharmacists are important members of that team. Second, pay attention! If Bev isn't with me at an appointment, I now take along a pen and paper to write down details so I don't forget.

When I asked my respirologist whether there were any new drugs for COPD, he said that he and others were actively researching a new long-acting bronchodilator that was similar to ipratropium. The new drug, called tiotropium, looked good in early tests, but even if the research continued to go well it would not likely be available for one to two years. I told him I would like to be one of the first to try it!

ARTHUR

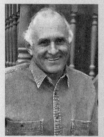

"I decided I didn't want to spend the rest of my life sitting in my living room watching *The Price Is Right*," says Arthur. "I'm too young to stop." So, drawing upon his natural strengths, he's become a planner *extraordinaire*.

Now fifty-six, Arthur was diagnosed with COPD in 1985. A technician with a pharmaceutical company in Montreal, he began to find it tough to climb the stairs at work. He'd arrive at the top, his chest heaving, get his air back, and light up a cigarette to calm down. "I figured once I quit smoking I'd get better, but I didn't," he recalls. "My wife's a nurse. She knew what was going on and she'd bring home articles on COPD for me to read. I'd read 'em, but it just didn't sink in." Bev finally persuaded him to visit a respirologist. "It's sunk in now," he says. "For me, it's all about ensuring it won't get any worse."

Having COPD has meant learning several important lessons. "I've learned that I have limits — and I stay within them," he begins. "Just because your friend can walk ten miles doesn't mean you can. I know what I can do and I do it. But the hardest lesson I learned was setting aside my pride." Bev nods in agreement.

Arthur spent his childhood working with his father in the dust of a cattle barn. He took up smoking at sixteen. Adult life revolved around his family, his sports, and his work. Devoted to his two sons, he coached their softball teams. "Summer was softball, winter was curling," remembers Arthur. That's changed.

Today, he's a walker. He spends his days strolling from his rural home to the local convenience store, where he finds a few neighbours to converse with over coffee. He and Bev discovered the pleasure of cruises and have travelled to Alaska, the Caribbean, and Florida. A collector, Saturdays he

We reviewed my oxygen saturation test (oximetry), which showed a saturation level of 94 percent at rest and 91 percent while walking, which provided reassurance that home oxygen was not necessary.

I also told my respirologist that I'd had my annual flu shot, and he said that was great, as the flu shot is one of the best ways to help stay infection-free over the winter. The respirologist said he'd phone my pharmacist with prescriptions — and repeats — for Oxeze, for the antibiotic I use if I have a lung infection, and for prednisone (the corticosteroid he wants me to take if I have a bad COPD flare-up). He advised me to stay away from crowds of people in the winter and from visitors with an obvious cold or the flu, since socializing is an easy way to pick up one of these bugs.

While we were discussing the winter season, I asked about my increasing difficulty with cold weather. He told me not to worry about it because my lung function was stable. He suggested that I wear a mask or scarf over my nose and mouth to warm the air slightly before it hits my lungs.

haunts local estate sales, scooping up bargains. And he's a photographer. Bev bought him a camera a few years back. He can't roughhouse with his grandkids, so Arthur has become the family photographer. He's also a singer. On Sundays you'll find Arthur performing in the choir of his church. Above all, he's a planner. Planning skills allow Arthur to fully enjoy all his new activities.

"I've always got a plan. I always think ahead," he explains. "That way I can avoid a flare-up in my breathing." Thinking ahead allows Arthur to quell his anxiety about the unknown and the unexpected challenges that could cause him to become short of breath. "I'll be anxious if I think there might be a challenge — a long walk at an airport, for example — and I haven't planned for it. It's the only thing I can think about. I get very worried about the unknown and I feel myself starting to breathe heavier and faster. But if I've planned for the situation — let's say I've called ahead to the airport and arranged for a wheelchair — I've eliminated the challenge, alleviated the anxiety, and my breathing stays under control. Planning allows me to do so many more things."

But it still bothers Arthur that he can't do his share of work around the house. This was a very sore point for Bev and Arthur for several years after his diagnosis. "I'm a nurse," explains Bev. "I'd like to do a little bit for everyone. When Arthur was diagnosed with COPD, my first inclination was to smother him with care. I did everything for him. That was wrong. It made me exhausted and Arthur was angry about feeling useless." The couple worked through this tough time by talking about their feelings. "I realized that I needed to let Arthur come forth with his suggestions and his ideas of how to deal with things," says Bev. "He's doing that now." Together, they've arrived at many compromises. For example, Arthur doesn't mow the lawn anymore (they've hired someone to do that) but he does all the dishes, something Bev used to do. "And," laughs Bev, "he talks a lot. He doesn't keep stuff inside. That's good for both of us."

He advised me not to become housebound, warning that it's all too easy to get out of shape if I stay inside all winter. Breathing is an endurance sport, he told me. That means staying in the best physical shape possible. He suggested equipping my boots with steel cleats that make it easier to walk on ice, so I won't become anxious about falling.

I reminded my respirologist that I have no choice about getting out of the house in the winter — I have several daily obligations. I sing in our church choir and a local barbershop group. In addition, I work every afternoon, helping my daughter-in-law, who has a business preparing soup mixes using dried beans. I help her sort the beans. The respirologist was very concerned about the quality of air in the barn where I work, suggesting that the dust from the beans could be a problem for me if the ventilation was inadequate. To date, I haven't had any problems with my breathing when I work, but we agreed that I'd start wearing a mask when I sort the beans.

My respirologist again mentioned the possibility of enrolling me in a local lung rehabilitation program. But when we both thought a bit more about it, we decided that I have a pretty good grasp of how to manage my COPD. I was keeping myself quite fit and at a good "playing weight." We figured the travel time a rehabilitation program would involve for me (I'd have to drive into Ottawa) might not make it worthwhile just now.

Then we discussed the winter escape Bev and I planned — our upcoming Caribbean cruise. My respirologist was concerned about the airline flight, explaining that oxygen levels are lower in airplanes despite pressurized cabins. Flying is equivalent to standing atop a 2,500-metre-high mountaintop — the air is thinner up there. He suggested that, before our trip, I return to the hospital for a test where low air pressure is simulated (like being in the cabin of a plane) — to see how my blood gases would manage. If I needed extra oxygen, he would help me make the necessary arrangements with the airline. He reminded me to take along adequate supplies of my drugs, including antibiotics and corticosteroids, just in case. When I returned for my flight simulation appointment, the respirologist would provide me with a letter to give to the ship's doctor, outlining my condition and the specifics of the drugs I take.

I'm hoping that, if I stick to our preventative maintenance plan, I won't see the respirologist again until next year — same time, same place.

BUILDING YOUR TEAM

COPD can affect all aspects of your life and the lives of your family. It's hard for any one person to know all the resources that are available to help you cope with COPD — and there are many. Managing COPD really is a team sport, so we've listed some of the people you may meet along the way, and some of the resources you can access on your own. Remember — you are not alone!

Who Are All These People and What Are They Doing to Me?

Let's say your family doctor thinks you have COPD and would like you to have some further testing done at the local hospital. Or maybe your respirologist thinks you're not eating right. Possibly your family is having difficulty coping with your special needs and you'd like to see what your options are for home care. COPD will take you into a new world of medical professionals. People who test you, counsel you, poke you, prod you, and help you cope with your COPD. But who are all these people and what are their responsibilities toward you and your COPD?

Primary Care Physician: You probably call your primary care physician your family doctor or your general practitioner. Your primary care physician will meet with you regularly and when you have special concerns about your health. In addition, he or she will supervise your tests, medications, and other treatment you require, and coordinate consultations with lung specialists when needed.

Clinic Nurse: The clinic nurse works together with your primary care physician and will often help with testing and treatments.

Respirologist: A respirologist specializes in diagnosing and treating disorders of the respiratory system, specifically the lungs. He or she treats patients with asthma, COPD, pulmonary fibrosis, pneumonia, and lung cancer — among other diseases. In the United States, these specialists are called pulmonologists and, in Quebec, pneumologistes.

Respiratory Therapist (RT): This therapist performs both diagnostic and therapeutic procedures. In other words, a respiratory therapist helps assess your lung problems by conducting breathing tests that measure the capacity and capabilities of your lungs (like your FEV_1). Plus, after the diagnosis, he or she may be involved in helping you think about exercising, stress management, and proper breathing techniques. The respiratory therapist is trained to help you make the lifestyle and physical conditioning changes that will help you better cope with your COPD. If you're prescribed supplemental oxygen, a respiratory therapist will help you learn how to use it and monitor your oxygen equipment. In Ontario, this therapist may also be called a registered respiratory care practitioner, or RRCP.

Physiotherapist: Physiotherapy involves treating diseases and injuries with massage, exercise, manipulation, and other methods rather than with drugs. This means that a physiotherapist will assess your physical needs and design a treatment to suit you. The treatment could involve breathing techniques, ways to control your cough, and methods of dealing with breathlessness, flare-ups, and lung infections. A physiotherapist can also teach you specific exercises to improve your physical condition and help clear your lungs of mucus more effectively.

Social Worker: A social worker helps people with special needs. For those with COPD, a social worker can provide counselling to help you and your family cope with the impact of your disease.

73

Depending on your circumstances, a social worker could help you find someone to come and help you in your home or, if necessary, he or she could assist you in finding a placement in a retirement residence or a nursing home. In addition, a social worker may be able to help you gain access to financial aid for things you might need, including oxygen and medications.

Dietician: A dietician, or nutritional consultant, can help you sort out issues relating to your diet. This includes assessing your nutritional needs and dealing with any problems you may be experiencing. A dietician can help you identify ways to meet your nutritional needs and can advise you on the types of foods you need and how to prepare them.

Psychologist: A psychologist specializes in those functions of the mind that affect human behaviour. COPD is a difficult and chronic disease that can radically change the life of anyone it affects, as well as the life of the caregiver or partner. These changes can create emotional difficulties, and a psychologist is trained to help you cope with these issues. A psychologist can counsel you and your caregiver in ways to cope with the stress and hardship you experience because of your COPD.

Occupational Therapist: Occupational therapists deal with many of the practical physical activities necessary for normal activities of daily living. An occupational therapist will help you become as independent as possible in your day-to-day activities. This may involve learning to simplify how you do things and how to conserve energy when performing daily chores like showering and dressing, or preparing meals and cleaning up.

Recreational Therapist: You might think a diagnosis of COPD means the end of fun in your life. You may have to give up favourite sports, for example. A recreational therapist can teach you otherwise, counselling you on ways to fill your leisure hours with new activities that match your physical abilities.

Pharmacist: The person who dispenses your drugs is also an expert source of information about those drugs, specifically how to administer them and any possible side effects. Get to know your pharmacist and make sure you ask for details about the drugs you are prescribed.

Hey, I Need Some Help Here!

You may not qualify for a formal rehabilitation program, or maybe you live in a community where there isn't a pulmonary rehab program. But you still have needs. How do you get them met? What if you think you need a walker? Where do you go? What if you're not sure whether you're eating properly and you'd like some guidance? What if you'd like to take a course to learn how to manage the stress of living with a chronic disease? What if you feel that you need some help around the house?

First and foremost, your needs will not be met unless you make them known. That means asking — loud and clear — for the help you feel you need. And if you feel you're not being well served by the first person or organization you speak to, approach another! In today's health care system, the meek do not inherit the earth.

Whom do you ask? Well, that depends on what you're looking for. Sometimes it's clear whom to approach. For example, if you think you might need supplemental oxygen, make an appointment with your doctor and, if it's discovered that you do, contact a local oxygen supplier. You can get names of oxygen suppliers from your doctor or by looking under "Oxygen" or "Oxygen Therapy Equipment" in your Yellow Pages.

Let's say you'd like to improve your physical condition. Again, the first stop will be your doctor's office to talk about what might work for you. If you live in a smaller community, there may not be an exercise class designed for people with COPD. You might end up working on a program designed for you by a physiotherapist. Or you might find an exercise program for seniors at your local community association. In this case, a copy of the Yellow Pages is a great place to start in your search for help with any issue relating to COPD.

Here's a general list of possible sources of information and help:

- **Your family doctor or respirologist** — Always the best place to start! Your doctor's nurse or secretary is also probably a fount of information.
- **The Lung Association** — For information on COPD, call The Lung Association's national toll-free information line at 1-888-566-LUNG (5864). Their Web site (www.lung.ca) has a comprehensive COPD section that includes an on-line version of the self-help program *Breathe Easy — A Program about Living with Lung Disease.*
- **Local hospitals** — Many hospitals offer access to rehabilitation programs or can help you find what you need in your community.
- **The public health unit of your municipality** — The public health unit may offer courses on a variety of topics and may also be able to direct you to other resources in your community. You'll find phone numbers in the Blue Pages of your phone book.
- **Local seniors' centres** — Offering courses on everything from tai chi to organizing your finances, seniors' centres can be a great source of information. Your local seniors' centre can probably help you with questions about pension entitlement and financial issues. COPD can be an expensive disease — you might need to pay for help around the house, for example — and your finances may become stretched. There may be public financial assistance programs available in your community for low-income or disabled seniors. If you are a veteran, contact Veterans Affairs of Canada (DVA). Similarly, you could probably get information at your local seniors' centre about community-based support services for seniors — everything from home repair to housekeeping to transportation services. Plus, seniors' centres offer opportunities to socialize, enjoyable outings, and interesting recreational activities.
- **The "Social and Human Service Organizations" listing in your Yellow Pages** — This listing is a treasure trove of information about services in your community. Not only does it include organizations with specific mandates like the Canadian Mental Health Association but it also lists community health centres. For example, in the Ottawa Yellow Pages, you'll find the number for the local Community Care Access Centre, a non-profit organization that provides home health care and support. This is the place Peg turned to when she needed a physiotherapist to get her started on an exercise program after her flare-up. Such organizations, funded by provincial governments, exist in many communities across Canada and provide a variety of services delivered by nurses, homemakers, occupational therapists, physiotherapists, nutritionists, and others.

- **The Ministry of Health of your province** — The provinces provide health care materials and also information about funding for treatments, oxygen, and assistive devices like walkers. You'll find phone numbers in the Blue Pages of your phone book.
- **Local community centres and the YM/YWCA** — The variety of courses offered by community centres and the YM/YWCA is amazing. These can be excellent places to join a yoga class, a support group, or a meditation program. Check them out!
- **Oxygen providers** — Even if you're not on oxygen, these companies can be good sources of information. Because they deal with people with chronic lung diseases all the time, they learn plenty about what's going on in the community. It was through the oxygen company Access Therapy, for example, that we learned about travel agencies that specialize in helping people with lung diseases.
- **The Red Cross** — The Red Cross offers many services, including homemaking services and Meals on Wheels. Phone the Red Cross in your community or check out their programs on the Internet at www.redcross.ca.
- **The Internet** — It's amazing what's out there in cyberspace. Type in a few key words (COPD, emphysema, lung disease) and you'll be overwhelmed by what turns up. Beware, however! Not all Internet sites are created equal. Some are reliable (The Lung Association's site, for example), some are not. Here are a few informative sites for COPD information: The Canadian Lung Association (www.lung.ca), the Colorado HealthSite (www.coloradohealthnet.org), the American Association for Respiratory Care (www.aarc.org), the National Jewish Medical and Research Center (www.njc.org), and the American Lung Association (www.lungusa.org). If you're not certain about the information your gather on the Internet, check it out with your doctor before acting upon it.
- **Other people with COPD** — These are the folks who are going through the same things you are. Why not pick their brains to see what they've learned along the way? The Lung Association in your community may operate a COPD support group where people can gather to exchange ideas.

6

High Anxiety — Riding the Emotional Roller Coaster of COPD

One simple story can give us a remarkable insight into how one person and his family are coping emotionally with the diagnosis of COPD. Similarly, one simple event can be a catalyst for positive emotional change. For Arthur and his wife, Bev, the story and the event concern a disability permit for the family car.

Fear, guilt, anger, anxiety, loneliness, and frustration are as much a part of COPD as breathlessness, fatigue, coughing, and spitting. Just ask Arthur. Arthur was always a "go for it" kind of guy — active in competitive sports and successful at a challenging and physically demanding job. A proud person, he delighted in a busy life full of family, work, sports, and volunteer activities. Then along came COPD. First, it was just a bit of breathlessness. He found he was relying on the other guys at work to do things he used to do. Then he started to struggle for breath while mowing the lawn. He figured giving up cigarettes would cure the situation. But quitting cold turkey didn't cure him. In fact, his breathlessness was becoming more pronounced. Arthur started to find walking any distance tough. When they'd drive somewhere, either Bev would drop him off at the door or they'd arrive extra early so that they'd get a spot close to the entrance.

When he was diagnosed with COPD, Arthur still thought he could beat it and return to his old active ways. He denied both the extent and the permanence of his disability. One symbol of that denial was his refusal to obtain a disability permit for the family car.

Bev recalls it this way: "At first, Arthur was Mr. Pride. He was only in his forties when he was diagnosed, and it was tough for both of us to adjust. He was angry. He was young; others his age were fine. It wasn't fair."

Arthur refused to get a disability permit allowing him parking privileges. Why would he want a permanent symbol on the dashboard of his car proclaiming his disability to the world? Bev, on the other hand, was tired of chauffeur duties and arriving hours before events started. She was also tired of Arthur's reluctance to acknowledge his disease to friends and family. Initially, Arthur didn't want people to know he was struggling. "Do you think people can't see what's happening?" Bev would ask him. "People can see you have to stop every few steps to get a few breaths." Bev took the issue into her own hands, obtaining a disability permit and arriving home with it prominently displayed in the car.

"We had a few short sentences," says Bev in her understated way. She had started to accept the changes Arthur's disease would mean for both of them. She wanted to acknowledge the change COPD created and get on with their lives. That argument was a turning point. It was time for Arthur to publicly acknowledge the change COPD had brought to their lives and to deal with his anger.

Arthur can look back now and admit that it took a long time for him to allow the fact of his COPD to sink in. But Bev realized she needed to change too. She now admits she had been smothering Arthur: "I'd say, 'Don't do that, I'll get it.' I realized I was bugging him to death. I needed to step back and let him come forth with his suggestions of how to deal with things." For Bev and Arthur, the argument over the permit served to clear the air between them, allowing them to think about their behaviours and beliefs — and set about changing them.

Over the years, they've worked together and adapted, altering their lives to accommodate what Arthur *can* do and trying not to dwell on what they've lost. It's been hard work for both of them, but, as Bev says, "If we don't do this, we're only going to compound our problems." They began to realize that although they may have lost ground in some areas, they had the opportunity to grow and gain much more as they met their new challenges together.

Arthur and Bev are lucky. They have a solid marriage and a warm relationship with their children and grandchildren. They're talkers who obviously enjoy one another's company. Between them, they've got a large collection of good friends and a wide variety of hobbies and interests. The result? They have an upbeat, realistic approach to life. But as the disability permit story illustrates, even they have had their emotional battles riding the COPD roller coaster.

With chronic illness comes stress. And stress takes an emotional and physical toll. Chronic disease changes you, limiting your life, affecting your family. We know that worry, anxiety, and stress can exacerbate breathing problems, particularly breathlessness.

We all live with stress in our lives. Each of us copes with it in our own unique way. Some keep their cool no matter what; others flip out at the drop of a hat. But no matter how good we are at coping, our bodies are not designed to deal with the continuous stress that a chronic disease places on them. Never-ending stress can literally wear out your body, weaken your immune system, and leave you susceptible to such problems as infections, memory lapses, depression, anxiety, and high blood pressure.

There are bad and good ways of coping with stress. If your habit of one or two glasses of wine each week has crept up to three or four each night, you've found a way to cope with COPD, but it's not a good one. Similarly, if you find you're now smoking more than ever before, you're coping, but not well. Focusing on things you can control in your life is one way to work toward returning your life to normal. The goal is to find ways to deal with your emotional problems that leave you (and those around you) both emotionally and physically stronger.

Getting Help — If You Need It

Most of us wouldn't think twice about seeking help for a physical problem. But emotional problems — even though they can cause physical problems in the long run — are a different matter. For many, admitting we need emotional help is akin to announcing we're crazy. We see it as a sign of weakness or failure — a loss of control.

Most people with COPD can benefit from learning coping skills to deal with the emotional challenges presented by COPD. And it's not just the person with COPD who can use some help; family members and even friends all face new challenges in dealing with the stress of COPD. And help is available to learn better ways of doing things and dealing with chronic illness. Help can come from within (from you and your family) and from without (experts skilled at aiding us find the support we need).

Your Family Doctor: Your doctor is a good place to start. Arrange a special meeting with your doctor and your family. Be sure to let the doctor know well in advance what you want to discuss so extra time can be set aside for the appointment. Do your homework first. Make a list of the topics you want to talk about. Let it all hang out! This is the time to get all your fears, anxieties, angers, and questions on the table. You may need several sessions to get a proper handle on how you, your family, and your doctor can best deal with the situation. Your doctor may use these sessions to determine whether you might benefit from some more formal support, such as the resources listed below.

Pulmonary Rehabilitation Programs: Many of the emotional support

---

JUST THINKING ABOUT BREATHLESSNESS MAKES ME BREATHLESS!

The condition of your body contributes to breathlessness. But what about the condition of your mind? Listen to Arthur. "I was getting ready to go to a funeral the other day. Getting my formal clothes together, being in a bit of a rush, I could feel myself becoming breathless and I knew I could start hyperventilating. When that happens, I find myself breathing much heavier from my chest, my breathing speeds up, my rib cage is working hard to expand. If it goes on for any length of time, I start getting lightheaded, my thoughts start coming rapidly, and my rib cage becomes extremely sore."

Arthur was stressed emotionally while preparing for the funeral: anxious about getting to the service on time, worried about how far the walk would be into the church, wondering how many stairs he'd have to tackle during the day. These emotional stressors caused a very real physical reaction. Arthur could feel himself becoming breathless. His anxiety contributed to heavier breathing, an increase in the volume of air he was taking in (difficult for Arthur given that his COPD has resulted in significant hyperinflation of his lungs), an increased use of oxygen, and an increase in the tension of his respiratory muscles. All of this physical work, in turn, started to increase his heart rate. It looked as if he'd get caught in the vicious cycle of anxiety culminating in an attack of breathlessness — a panic attack.

On this day, Arthur was able to nip the anxiety/breathlessness cycle in the bud. "When I feel

---

services that can help improve coping skills can be found as part of a comprehensive pulmonary rehabilitation program. (See chapter 7 for more information.)

Support Groups: Support groups, composed of people with COPD, are a great place to learn how others are coping with the disease. You'll hear what works for others and how they go about their daily lives. And you'll learn you're not the only one living with COPD. By "normalizing" your condition, you'll learn to cope better. These groups, often organized under the auspices of The Lung Association, have interesting names, like the "Huff and Puffers" or the "S.O.B. (Shortness of Breath) Club." The groups often work best when they include an exercise component. The group setting helps to maintain motivation for the self-directed pulmonary rehabilitation that is so essential for coping with the burdens imposed by both aging and COPD. Sometimes these groups encourage family members to attend sessions. Contact The Lung Association in your area if you're interested in joining a COPD support group.

Individual Counselling: One-on-one counselling sessions with a therapist can help you tackle specific issues, including stress, anxiety, or depression. If you feel you need individual help, ask your family doctor to

breathlessness coming on," he explains, "I start talking to myself. 'Sit down, relax, wait a bit until you've calmed down.' I sat down on the edge of the bed, counted to fifty, practised pursed-lip breathing. I probably sat there for about two or three minutes, collecting myself and my thoughts. Once my breathing was under control, I got myself ready. I was fine the rest of the day." (See the sidebar "Don't Panic — SOS Breathing for SOB (Shortness of Breath)" in chapter 7 for more information on breathing exercises and panic attacks.)

Arthur advises thinking ahead — identify situations that could cause emotional stress (one person's stressor may not cause stress for another) and then deal as slowly and calmly as you can with that situation. For Arthur, breaking down tasks is one way to avoid emotional stress. For example, when getting ready for an emotional outing like a funeral, "I put on my shoes and then sit down for a bit, I put my coat on and then wait a minute or two. I avoid getting myself worked up. Then I hope like hell that the car is parked near the door!"

Communicating these anxieties is a good way to start coping with them. Your family needs to know your emotional triggers so they can be avoided or mitigated. You might also consider a support group of others with COPD where you'd learn from the experiences of others how to cope emotionally. Also consider behavioural therapy — relaxation techniques or biofeedback. Speak to your doctor or contact your local chapter of The Lung Association.

recommend a therapist, preferably someone familiar with respiratory problems and chronic illness. You can usually arrange for counselling through a pulmonary rehabilitation program.

Group Counselling: Like support groups, group counselling brings together people suffering from respiratory problems. These group sessions are led by a trained therapist with the goal of helping you gain control of your illness and learn effective coping strategies. Speak to your doctor or contact The Lung Association to locate a group in your community.

Family Counselling: No one is an island. The issues you're experiencing with your COPD will inevitably spill over into your family. Just as you may have problems coping with COPD, so might your family members. Family counselling, led by a trained therapist, can teach family members to talk openly about their concerns and problems, which is the first step to solving them. This is often best done by therapists with experience with COPD, such as those linked to a pulmonary rehabilitation program.

Psycho-educational Groups: These groups are targeted at specific issues — quitting smoking, controlling alcohol, managing stress, learning to relax. Depending on the issue you wish to address, consider contacting The Lung Association, your local YM/YWCA, neighbourhood community centres, or Alcoholics Anonymous.

Spiritual Support: Although there's no scientific proof that prayer can heal, believers tell us their faith, combined with support from members of their religious community, provides emotional stability, serenity, and hope. For many, meditation and prayer serve to relax both body and soul. Speak to your clergy person about programs offered in your community.

Tai Chi and Yoga: Many people develop great physical and emotional comfort from practising disciplines such as tai chi or yoga. Both aim to link emotional and spiritual energy with physical energy. And in doing so, both can improve breathing, muscle strength, and flexibility, while relaxing both body and mind. Both are good for people who, because of their respiratory limitations, can't do aerobic exercises. Contact your local YM/YWCA or health club. If you prefer the privacy of your home, plenty of instructional videos and books are available on both yoga and tai chi.

Reaction of Family and Friends

"Man's Care for His Disabled Wife Does More Harm Than Good." This recent headline ran atop a Dear Abby column concerning a husband who did everything for his disabled wife, confining her to bed and controlling her life, rather than encouraging her to be as independent as possible. In suggesting that both the husband and wife needed emotional support, Abby explained that situations like these aren't unusual.

Family members tend to fall between two extremes: overkill (like the husband in the Dear Abby column) or dismissal ("You're not sick! Pull up your socks!"). Louise's family fell closer to the "dismissal" end of the spectrum. "At the beginning, my husband and daughter didn't know what to expect. They didn't know how sick I was, and they honestly thought I'd get better. Looking back, I think they were in denial. They hoped I'd get better, so they tried to minimize what I was going through. We hit a turning point when I went on round-the-clock oxygen. We talked a lot and I told them, 'I'm not going to get better. I'm really limited now.'"

Once she'd explained her situation, Louise and her husband set about negotiating. "We worked out a deal between us that lets me do as much as I'm able. For example, he cooks and I do cleanup on the condition that the dishes get done when I feel up to it. So our dinner dishes might not get washed until the next morning. Who cares? It works for us."

But there's more to this deal than just housekeeping chores. When Louise tells her husband, Deac, that she is able to do something, she means it and he listens. Similarly, when she says she's incapable of tackling a chore or event, he respects that too. They try to be very honest with one another about their abilities and feelings. For the most part, their routine works for them.

Louise is smart to keep plugging away at household chores rather than leaving them all to Deac. Breathing is, after all, an endurance sport, and working around the house is one way to keep physically active. That's why family members in "overkill" mode are doing no favours for their loved ones with COPD. By taking on all the responsibilities of the person with COPD, they are reducing that individual to a helpless, childlike state. They figure if they do all the cleaning and other chores, their disabled loved one will get better, or at least not get worse. Again, this is a situation where the caregiver needs education. When it comes to lungs, use them or lose them. Encouraging a person with COPD to adopt a sedentary lifestyle is a sure way to worsen his or her condition.

Like you, your family members will cope much better if they too learn to live with all aspects of COPD — everything from practical issues (you can't keep the house as clean as you'd like) to the emotional (fear of premature disability or death). Pulmonary rehabilitation programs often offer family group meetings to aid in the coping process. If there are no formal rehabilitation resources in your area, arrange a group meeting with your family and your family doctor. Other options for family counselling may be available in your community.

Getting On with Your Life

COPD is a disease of loss. As lung function is lost, so is the ability to do many of the things that once provided pleasure. Arthur, for example, no longer plays baseball, curls, or gardens. Edgar can't participate in martial arts. Jean is now unable to hike through her beloved countryside. It's easy to become overwhelmed by these losses, chronically unhappy, irritable, angry, and even clinically depressed. Isolation, loneliness, and social withdrawal are natural products of an unhappy personality. How do you get on with your life when everything's changed — forever?

Then there's the reaction of family and friends. They may not understand or appreciate the losses that accompany your condition. Unlike other diseases, COPD doesn't ravage your body outwardly — it simply takes away your breath. To those around you, you may look the same. Your losses may not be visible, but they're still very real. People might trivialize your loss: "So you can't play baseball anymore. So what! You're still alive, aren't you? Pull yourself together and don't feel sorry for yourself." Or they might suggest you should feel guilty for causing your illness: "What did you expect? Think of all the cigarettes you smoked!"

An essential element of living with a chronic illness is recognizing that it will be with you for the rest of your life. You won't be able to go back to baseball, martial arts, or hikes through the countryside. Those elements of your life are lost to you. To adapt to those profound losses, begin by grieving for them. Just like you'd grieve for a friend who died, grieve for your losses. Once you've worked through the grieving process, it will be time to move on, adapt, and find new challenges and activities.

It's important to recognize that you've lost important pieces of yourself that once helped define you. If you're going to adapt to your new state, you must first recognize those losses. Recognition won't occur overnight. Look at Arthur's experience. He couldn't come to grips with his loss of mobility. It wasn't until Bev came home with a disability permit that he began to recognize and accept his loss.

An integral part of the recognition process is identifying and eliminating harmful emotions that may be impeding your ability to deal with your disease. Guilt is one of the biggies. Peg refers to her COPD as her "self-inflicted wound." Take that too seriously and you might not seek the help you need because you feel you don't deserve it. Hindsight is 20/20. You didn't intend to develop COPD but you've got it now and guilt isn't going to change a thing. Nip guilt in the bud. If it's impeding the way you manage your disease, talk to your partner or your family doctor or get help from a therapist.

Once you've accepted your losses, it's time to deal with the emotions attached to them. Working through the sadness or anger you feel because you can no longer garden or cross-country ski or ride a bike is a tall order. This is where you can use support — a friend, a family member, a spiritual adviser, maybe even a professional therapist or support group. We're raised to be self-sufficient and to place a high value on being "in control" of our emotions. It's hard to accept that often we can't do it all alone. When a chronic illness like COPD profoundly affects our lives, asking for and accepting help can be very tough but, perhaps surprisingly, very rewarding.

Experimenting with alternatives to your old activities is a natural next step. Mychelle provides a couple of examples. She can no longer bike during the summers, so she's taken up golf. Cross-country skiing winds her, so now she downhill skis. Louise has discovered books, movies, Broadway shows, and COPD exercise classes. Arthur has developed a passion for photography and antiquing. All are quick to admit that these activities are not substitutes for their former ones. They acknowledge that they've entered a new phase of their lives — one filled with new and different activities.

Mychelle, Arthur, and Louise have moved on. They haven't allowed themselves to become stuck grieving for their losses. By recognizing their losses, dealing with the emotions attached to those losses, experimenting with alternatives, and, finally, forming attachments to new activities, they've succeeded in getting on with their lives.

It sounds easy when it's summarized in a couple of paragraphs. Mychelle, Arthur, and Louise are a resourceful trio, naturally good copers who have always filled their lives with plenty of diverse activities. Not everyone is as well rounded. Remember, there's no shame in getting help or in talking to someone about your emotional issues.

Dealing with Your Fears

"If you can't breathe, you're frightened," says Peg. "You can't understand that kind of fear unless you've experienced it. You feel so helpless." Sometimes breathlessness gets out of control and starts to feed on itself, making you breathe faster, which leads to more breathlessness and more fear — which begets more breathlessness. Pretty soon, you panic. Breathlessness-induced panic attacks are not uncommon in people with COPD who have not learned the art of controlled breathing and relaxation. These are essential skills to learn. Chapters 7 and 8 give details on dealing with panic attacks.

If you can't breathe, fear is a completely normal reaction. That's why it's so important to work with your doctor or therapist to learn how to get your breathing under control.

But there's a point where your fear can become fear of fear itself. Because you're afraid of becoming breathless, you stop doing things. To avoid the anxiety that accompanies your COPD, you find you're sitting at home, doing nothing. The trick lies in figuring out which are rational fears and which are irrational and the degree to which irrational fears are making you avoid the things you're afraid of, causing you distress, or impairing your life. A good place to start is with a thorough understanding of breathlessness. Yes, it might be embarrassing to suffer a bout of breathlessness in a shopping mall but, hey, it's not going to kill you. If your fear of breathlessness is keeping you from doing things, maybe it's time to deal with that anxiety and develop some new coping skills.

You'll be surprised how helpful it is to talk about your fears rather than keeping them to yourself. Support groups are a great place to learn how others cope. Anxiety can also be treated with relaxation therapies such as biofeedback, and exercise programs, including breathing exercises. A therapist can help you deal with the thinking that accompanies your anxiety and find specific ways to change it. You can also speak to your doctor about anti-anxiety drugs and the other measures to control breathlessness discussed in chapter 10.

And don't forget your family. They deserve the right to help you with your COPD. There's no place for false bravado here. Maybe you are used to being the "big cheese" in the family, but now is the time to learn the essential art of being humble. Ask someone you love for help. By acknowledging that you are mortal, you'll often be able to reopen doors in your life that have practically closed.

Dragged Down by Depression

Janet talks about her many losses, most caused by COPD. She lost her job as a nurse and can't do many of the things she once loved. Many of her friends left her life because she was unable or unwilling to both sustain the friendships and cope with her disease. She's worried she might be forced to sell her house because she can no longer maintain it. She can't do it herself and she can't afford to hire someone. She admits she's lonely and worried. She's a perfect candidate for depression.

Chronic illness is a common cause of depression. People with chronic illness often feel helpless in the face of a disease that has no cure. In fact, COPD patients may be at increased risk for depression. Many smokers unconsciously rely on nicotine as an antidepressant. Once cigarettes are gone from their lives — in combination with a diagnosis of COPD — depression may enter. This is one of the reasons why nicotine replacement therapy and bupropion (an antidepressant medication) work so well in assisting smoking cessation.

The Canadian Mental Health Association provides good information on depression and its treatment. Here is their checklist of the signs that a person might be suffering from depressive illness:

— feeling worthless, helpless, or hopeless
— sleeping more or less than usual
— eating more or less than usual
— having difficulty concentrating or making decisions
— loss of interest in taking part in activities
— decreased sex drive
— avoiding other people
— overwhelming feelings of sadness or grief

— feeling unreasonably guilty
— loss of energy, feeling very tired
— thoughts of death or suicide

If you have been experiencing any of these symptoms, it may be time to seek professional help. Start by speaking to your family doctor. It may also help to ask your doctor to check your blood oxygen levels. If you've developed chronic hypoxemia, depression-like symptoms may be a sign.

Because of the stigma surrounding depressive illness, many people wait too long before getting the treatment they need. And help is available in the form of counselling and medication. Family, friends, and support groups can play a big role in helping a sufferer recover from depression.

For more information about depression, contact your local branch of the Canadian Mental Health Association. Check their Web site at www.cmha.ca or call their headquarters in Toronto at (416) 484-7750.

JANET

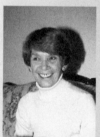

"These guys keep me going," says Janet, picking up one of the four Pekingese dancing at her feet. "I know my breathing would be better if I didn't have four dogs — and all of their hair — in the house. But I need them. They give me the extra push I need to get on with things. And I definitely would not want to walk into an empty house." So she's made her choice. It's a choice that gives her a set, predictable routine — starting with a daily vacuuming ritual.

For Janet, COPD is as much a disease of the head as the lungs. "There are so many things I'd like to be doing — volunteer work, for example. But I'm nervous that I'll get myself worked up, and once I get anxious that affects my breathing. I know that's not COPD. That's just me — I can get myself into a real tizzy!" So Janet has turned her attention to her "babies." "They keep me really active," she says.

COPD has been a disease of frustration for Janet. Always competent and in charge, Janet, now sixty-five, was a nurse for nearly thirty years until her retirement in 1989. She raised four children single-handedly after her divorce in the late 1960s. "I was so used to doing what I wanted when I wanted to do it," she says. "I can't do that anymore. Plus, I'm watching my skills diminish before my eyes. Last year, I had to give up shovelling the snow from the driveway. I was barely able to wash and wax my car this summer. I won't be able to do that next summer. Watching my own deterioration is so frustrating for me."

So what is she doing to handle her frustration? She learned early on that she needed to talk to someone who understood how she was feeling. "I felt embarrassed in front of many of my old friends

— what with my coughing and huffing and puffing. I felt like an outcast. Mind you, I never sat down with them and explained what COPD was all about. I regret that today. But I did join a support group at the local branch of The Lung Association — the S.O.B. (Shortness of Breath) Club. We meet twice weekly to exercise, have a cup of tea with cookies, and a chat. Socializing with your own kind is very good for me. We're all different but we have the same problems. I feel comfortable there.

"I was a nurse for years but I've learned that I still have so much to learn about this disease," she continues. "And the most important thing I've learned is the need to keep active. I need exercise. When I was first diagnosed, I cut out walking. I figured if I could just sit still my breathing would be okay. But it wasn't."

Janet was shocked by the suddenness of the onset of her COPD. "I thought COPD was a disease that crept up on you slowly. I got out of bed one morning in the winter of 1991 and thought: 'Gee, I can't breathe.' During the day, my condition worsened. I went to my family doctor, who diagnosed a lung infection, which he treated with antibiotics. From then on, I was constantly battling bronchitis and lung infections. I went from good health to chronic illness virtually overnight." By 1992, her family doctor had prescribed a bronchodilator. Her breathlessness continued to increase, and in 1996 her doctor referred her to a respirologist.

She's meticulous about food, ensuring that she eats a healthy, balanced diet. To look at her, however, you might wonder whether she eats at all. Janet is skinny. "I've always been tiny," she says. "But with COPD, I find I must eat small amounts several times each day. It chokes me if I have a large meal. I've found a few restaurants around town where I can order half-portions."

Janet works diligently at controlling her breathing. She's a convert to diaphragmatic breathing, which she learned in a rehabilitation program in 1999. She finds she can now bring more air into her lungs. And she is careful to use pursed-lip breathing whenever she tackles tough housecleaning activities — like cleaning up after her pups.

7

"Just Do It!" — The Importance of Pulmonary Rehabilitation

"When my family doctor first told me about a pulmonary rehabilitation program, I didn't know what he was talking about," begins Audrey. "It was at a hospital in the east end of Ottawa, and I live in the west end, so I didn't want to be bothered. 'Why would you want me to go way out there?' I asked him. 'I think it would do you good. Please go for the assessment at least and find out whether they'll let you enrol,' he told me. Well, I tried it. I was terrified the first day I started. But I didn't stop. In the end, the rehab program was great for me. It's been nearly five years since I graduated and I've kept up with my exercises — I now work out twice each week at Access Therapy, a local pulmonary exercise maintenance program, and I do exercises at home — every day, faithfully."

Audrey's experience isn't unusual. Like most patients with COPD, she was unaware that a formal pulmonary rehabilitation program existed in her community, and she didn't have a clue what went on in the program and why it might prove useful for her. Her initial response was a firm "no, thank you." When she did agree to attend, her first day in the program was marked by terror. Finally, however, she reaped the benefits. "I *feel* better and I *cope* better than I did before rehab."

90

Pulmonary rehabilitation programs like the one Audrey attended are offered in larger centres across North America. Typically based in hospitals, these programs take a comprehensive approach, focusing on educating patients about COPD and about exercise, nutrition, and coping skills — all with the goal of helping them better manage both life and COPD. To do this, these programs bring together a team of health care professionals, ranging from dieticians to physiotherapists to pharmacists to psychologists to social workers to physicians.

Not everyone lives in places where full-scale pulmonary rehab programs are available *and* not everyone with COPD needs to attend a comprehensive rehab program in the first place. Rest assured that there are plenty of alternatives available, ranging from the exercise maintenance program Audrey now attends, to more informal programs associated with smaller hospitals, to nutrition classes at your local community centre. Plus, many people with COPD have developed their own self-directed rehab programs, including activities they pursue on their own, often in their homes. We'll discuss all of these alternatives in this chapter. You'll find lots of practical tips for taking care of yourself in the final portion of the chapter, which deals with self-directed rehab programs.

Before we get into the details of what rehab programs provide, let's look at why you need them in the first place, starting with Audrey's story. Before her COPD manifested itself, Audrey was an active woman, caring for her children and travelling around the world in her career. But she'd never found much time for physical exercise. Then along came COPD, crashing into her life with a bout of pneumonia in 1992. Everything changed. Her husband became her caregiver. Very attentive, he ensured that she didn't have to lift a finger around the house. She could sit and rest. Sure enough, she became even less physically active than she'd been before the onset of COPD. She found herself troubled by phlegm accumulating in her lungs. No matter how much she coughed, she felt she could never get her lungs cleared out properly or completely. Then came the vicious cycle of hospitalizations. Audrey just couldn't stay away, landing in hospital up to five times each winter with various ailments all related to COPD: bouts of pneumonia, influenza, and bronchitis.

Audrey didn't realize it, but she was trapped in a downward spiral of inactivity sometimes referred to as the "down escalator" of COPD. Her physical abilities were dwindling, making her less likely or able to tackle new physical tasks. Her inactivity was leading to ever more inactivity. This was tough on her body, reducing both her cardiac fitness and the efficiency of the muscles in her arms and legs. In the end she felt lousy — fatigued, short of breath, and unhappy about her lack of independence and control. And she knew that her COPD wasn't going away, which made her feel even worse.

Her doctor knew that if Audrey continued along this path, she'd keep landing in hospital with acute flare-ups of her COPD. That cycle would end up increasing her level of disability. And if repeated flare-ups didn't do it, her increasingly sedentary lifestyle surely would. Plus, he knew Audrey's potential. He knew the woman who valued her independence and thrived on challenge. So he referred her to the Respiratory Rehabilitation Service at Ottawa's Rehabilitation Centre. (This is the normal process with most formal pulmonary rehabilitation programs. You need a referral from your doctor to begin the process.)

What could rehab offer Audrey? We know that once you've got COPD,

AUDREY

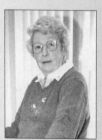

As Audrey walks the treadmill, she's talking quietly with a member of her respiratory maintenance program. They're in the sunny exercise room of an Ottawa oxygen therapy centre and they're discussing travel plans. "I've learned to pack the day before," she says to her companion. "If I have my luggage sitting beside the front door the night before I leave, I stay so much calmer."

The early 1990s were rough years for Audrey's health. In 1992 she began to notice breathing difficulties while preparing for Christmas and she landed in hospital with pneumonia in mid-December. That hospital admission was the first of many over the next two years. Audrey was in and out of the hospital up to five times each year with pneumonia and lung infections. Finally, in 1994, she was hospitalized for ten days. During that hospitalization, doctors diagnosed COPD.

Audrey found she was adopting an increasingly sedentary lifestyle at home. Her family doctor was blunt, telling her she needed to learn how to maintain her health, stay out of hospital, and regain her independence around the home. In 1995 she started a two-month rehabilitation program. She's been in the hospital only twice since then.

Appearances can be deceiving. Sitting still, Audrey looks the picture of health at age seventy-three. She is a beautiful, serene woman, soft spoken and gentle in her manner. But she's a "steel magnolia." While her four children were still in school, she began working as a typist in the government. Within six months, she was in charge of organizing international trade conferences around the world. She finished you've got it for keeps. Rehab can't boost your FEV_1 or improve your lung function in any other way. So what's the point?

Well, there's a lot more to COPD than FEV_1, and a rehab program is designed to maintain and enhance the quality of your life. It's clearly established that a rehab program can deliver:

— an improved capacity for exercise, which in turn improves mobility, endurance, and overall quality of life,
— a reduction in your breathlessness,
— an improvement in your ability to use your medications, specifically your inhalers, and
— an improved ability to cope with breathlessness and other restrictions imposed by COPD.

But there's more. The education and counselling you receive at rehab can give you more self-confidence and self-reliance and so may help keep

her career running the constituency office of a local member of Parliament. When the M.P. retired in 1988, he asked Audrey to join him working in the private sector. She chose retirement. "I told him I needed a breather." She chuckles now at the irony of that comment.

Throughout it all, she smoked. "I started when my first baby was six months old. We lived in a tiny apartment and rented a room to a woman. She got me started, asking me to sit down with her in the evening for a cigarette and a coffee." She smoked her final cigarette on December 6, 1993.

Audrey is certain of that date because it's marked in her diary. She carries the small book with her always. In it, she's noted all the salient details about the course of her disease — dates of hospitalizations, medications, details about her rehabilitation therapy (the degree of incline of the treadmill, for example). She charts the state of her breathing every day, together with the incidental happenings in her life. She relies on her diary to tell her if she's working toward a flare-up. Before she visits her doctor, she reviews her diary to check for trends in her condition and to formulate questions and requests. And she takes the diary with her to appointments to help her answer any questions doctors might have about the details of her health.

Audrey credits rehabilitation therapy with helping her live with COPD. "The exercises and breathing techniques definitely helped me," she says. She's faithfully followed an exercise regimen for the past five years. In addition to her twice-weekly maintenance exercise program at the oxygen therapy centre, she exercises at home every day. But the most important lesson for Audrey was probably the simplest. "I don't rush," she states emphatically. "It took me a while to learn that lesson. I can't charge into a store and back out like I used to. If I don't rush, there's still plenty of air left in me."

THE VICIOUS CYCLE OF BREATHLESSNESS

FIGURE 7.1: THE VICIOUS CYCLE
OF BREATHLESSNESS

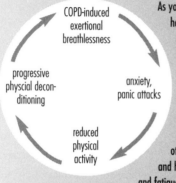

As you've already learned, breathlessness in COPD can have several causes, including narrowing of the airways, poor lung function leading to hypoxemia, hyperinflation, and weak muscles (breathing muscles and/or the muscles of your arms and legs). People with COPD tire very easily. That fatigue may be because of muscle weakness related to inactivity and to aging, in addition to the extra work of breathing imposed by COPD itself. But other coexisting illness, for example, arthritis, anemia, and heart disease, can also contribute to breathlessness and fatigue and should also be dealt with by your doctor.

Breathlessness in COPD can be categorized using a simple numeric scale:

0 — able to walk as far as you like on level ground, and to climb two flights of stairs without stopping
1 — unable to hurry or walk up hills or two flights of stairs without stopping
2 — unable to keep up with someone your own age at an ordinary pace on level ground
3 — unable to walk at your own pace without stopping
4 — unable to walk more than one block at a slow pace
5 — confined to house because of breathlessness

Obviously, on this test, the lower the score the better. Most people with level 3 or greater have an FEV_1 of less than 30 percent of predicted. There are, however, many people whose FEV_1 is higher than 30 percent who are nevertheless quite disabled by breathlessness. Others are able to maintain a high activity level despite a very low FEV_1. For these reasons, we often use other "end points" in COPD therapy — such as trying to quantify and improve a person's overall health or quality of life. That's where rehab — particularly learning to exercise properly — comes in.

Because of breathlessness and fatigue, many people with COPD have a tendency to drift into sedentary lifestyles that, not surprisingly, lead to further general and cardiovascular deconditioning, worsening symptoms, and diminishing overall health and quality of life. Frankly, it's depressing to be "lazy" because of weight gain and forced inactivity, to be unable to get out and enjoy life, and especially to have acquired such a fear of breathlessness that avoidance of normal activity becomes a way of life. It's crucial to try to break out of the vicious cycle of breathlessness leading to inactivity leading to more breathlessness . . .

you out of hospital when flare-ups occur and improve your overall health. In fact, rehab delivered all of those things, and more, for Audrey. Let's take a look at what you can expect from different types of rehab programs.

The Formal Pulmonary Rehabilitation Program

Typically, you must be referred to a rehab program by your doctor. If your doctor hasn't mentioned the possibility to you and you're interested, bring it up at your next appointment. Even if your doctor agrees to refer you, though, it's no guarantee of acceptance into the program. You'll be assessed to determine whether you're a good candidate for what the program has to offer. It may be that you're too ill, or that you're functioning at such a competent level already that the program can't offer you much. There are other considerations. In Ottawa, for example, you must have not smoked for a period of at least three months to be considered for admission.

Audrey, who was accepted into Ottawa's program in 1995, is probably the best one to walk us through a formal pulmonary rehabilitation program and tell us what it has to offer.

It's a blowy, cold day in February, five years after Audrey's first rehab experience, and she's returning for a visit and to renew acquaintances. Audrey won't hear of being dropped off at the door of Ottawa's Rehabilitation Centre; she insists on walking from the parking lot. "That's one of the things they taught me at rehab — I know my limits. I know that I can walk from the parking lot. I know how to pace myself. I'll stop and catch my breath if I need to. A little bit of breathlessness isn't the end of the world."

Once inside, she's joined by Colleen Kenney, the nurse educator for the program. "Oh boy, this brings back memories," Audrey says, looking around the hallways. The Ottawa program, currently headed by Dr. Douglas McKim, is offered on both an outpatient and inpatient basis. The outpatient program, which usually runs for about an hour twice weekly for eight to twelve weeks, is the one Audrey was enrolled in. It's the typical choice for patients who live in the Ottawa area and have moderate or mild COPD. Patients with more serious illness or who come from far away are admitted to the four-week inpatient program.

Approximately 170 COPD patients enroll in the Ottawa program each year, making it one of the largest in Canada. Together with Dr. McKim, Colleen assesses the patients and, based on the condition and needs of each patient, designs an individual program of exercise and education

---

WHAT A FORMAL REHABILITATION PROGRAM CAN DELIVER

Referral to a pulmonary rehabilitation program can be of great benefit for those who have become physically deconditioned, malnourished, or fearful of physical activity, and especially for those who could use some help with coping skills or are subject to panic attacks brought on by breathlessness. Such programs offer comprehensive approaches to pulmonary rehabilitation. With their multidisciplinary resources, they can focus on the five key elements of rehabilitation:

1. physical rehabilitation,
2. nutritional therapy,
3. education,
4. psychotherapy, and
5. counselling.

The potential benefits of comprehensive pulmonary rehabilitation include the following:

Physiotherapy/Exercise/Muscle Training
- improves and maintains skeletal and respiratory muscles as COPD advances
- permits increased exertional endurance with less breathlessness
- aids in clearance of bronchial secretions by teaching effective cough techniques
- helps control breathlessness by teaching effective relaxation techniques, pursed-lip breathing, and efficiency of movement in activities of daily living
- may reduce the need for hospitalization during COPD flare-ups
- helps people with COPD keep themselves mentally and physically active

Nutritional Counselling
As excessive weight loss or gain can worsen symptoms in COPD, nutritional counselling that promotes appropriate weight loss or nutritional supplementation to build up the breathing muscles can significantly improve symptoms in COPD.

Adjustment Therapy and Education
- teaches coping skills, stress management, emergency situation management, and the ability to deal with panic attacks
- helps with end-of-life decision planning

When successful, a multidisciplinary approach to pulmonary rehabilitation can considerably enhance overall health and life quality for people with advanced COPD, despite a lack of measurable improvement in FEV_1 or other aspects of lung function.

with the goal of increasing physical fitness and helping the patient live as normal a life as possible while coping with COPD.

Colleen and Audrey stroll into the respiratory lab. It's old-home week when Terry, the clinic nurse, and Kathy, the respiratory therapist, see Audrey at the door. (Because Audrey came down with a serious case of pneumonia during her participation in the program, she ended up taking nine months to finish her stint, graduating in the fall of 1995. "No wonder they remember me," she chuckles. "I'm sure they thought I'd never leave!")

Audrey's condition was assessed and tested during her time in the program, plus she returned for three follow-up visits (at three, six, and twelve months). In addition, Audrey has kept in contact with Terry over the years. Terry encourages former participants to phone her with any questions they have about continuing the rehab process on their own — new or different exercises, new programs in the community, that sort of thing. "It's reassuring to have a phone resource that's always open to me," says Audrey.

Audrey wasn't so calm when she first walked into this lab years ago and was subjected to the full range of testing, from pulmonary function tests to stress tests to cardiograms. "I was scared, and I was worried that, with all the testing, they'd find something even more serious than COPD. And everything seems even tougher when you're not feeling very well in the first place," she recalls.

Right from the outset, however, Audrey started to learn more about her disease. The rehab staff reviewed her medications with her, asking her to show them how she used her puffers. Then they worked with her, correcting and refining her techniques using the inhalers. The tests — and their results — were explained to her in detail. Just knowing more seemed to help in itself. The results were then sent along to the physiotherapists, who analyzed the extent of the limitation imposed on Audrey by her COPD and tailored an exercise program to her abilities.

Colleen and Audrey walk over to the physiotherapy room. "When I first came into this room, I thought: 'Good gracious! What do all these machines do? How will I ever do this? And what will this torture do for me anyway?'" She laughs at the memory.

The physiotherapy room is crowded with machines, including high-tech treadmills and stationary bikes. Plus, there are two three-way mirrors —

the kind you see in a dress shop — with stools in front of them. The walls are decorated with slogans ("Slow and Steady Wins the Race"), announcements ("Rehab Walking Club meets every Thursday"), drawings depicting exercises, and posters showing the target zone for heart rate. Several people are exercising. It's an active scene of organized confusion.

Audrey watches. "The first time I used these machines, I kind of freaked out. My blood pressure went up and I couldn't catch my breath. I really scared myself. But Maria Watson — she was my physiotherapist — convinced me to slow down and to continue, to get back on the stationary bike and try again. By the end of the program, I'd learned to control my breathing better while exercising. No more panic attacks."

Maria was able to persuade Audrey to get back on the machines after her initial scare by explaining that one of the benefits of a hospital-based rehab program is careful and complete monitoring of the health of the patient. Because the patient's heart rate and oxygen levels can be closely watched, she can push patients to their optimum and maximum level of activity, something that should not be done without proper monitoring.

Although physiotherapists work together with patients during the rehab program, one of the main goals of the exercise program is independence. Maria wants to give her patients confidence that they can keep their breathing under control while exercising, that they don't need to have a physiotherapist around all the time. Maria points to the stools by the mirrors. They're posture stools, she explains. Poor posture — with shoulders tensed up or slouched over — leads to increased shortness of breath. She works hard, exercising her patients' muscles to improve their posture. These "sitting exercises" are performed in front of the mirrors. "That way," explains Maria, "the patients can see what they're doing and repeat it at home themselves — because I can't go home with them!"

Audrey recalls her posture lessons. "I now work at keeping my shoulders down — not hunched up. There's a simple trick to help you do that — when you're sitting, you keep your palms turned up in your lap. That way, you don't put them flat on your knees which has the effect of raising your shoulders and making you use your accessory muscles." She's talking about the muscles that run from the neck to the collarbone. Overreliance on these muscles leads to poor posture that, in turn, increases shortness of breath. Maria's posture stool exercises focus on strengthening the breathing muscles you want working for you: the diaphragm (the breathing muscle underneath your lungs) and the intercostal muscles (small muscles between your ribs).

But it's not only the breathing muscles that are worked in this program. The heart muscle works together with the muscles of the arms and legs to power the body. The more efficiently all these muscles work, the more work they can do with less oxygen, which is a good thing for people with COPD, who may suffer from a lack of oxygen. Stronger muscles mean your heart doesn't have to work as hard or beat as fast to pump the same amount of blood. More power with fewer breaths!

Audrey watches a woman exercising her arms on a stationary bike. "When you're working on your arms and legs, you're working on very different muscles. If you try to work both at the same time, it can get confusing and you can become very short of breath. So we worked them separately." The arm muscles are often the easiest to forget. You don't often exercise them, yet they're really important. If you've got COPD, your chest muscles can use all the help they get from strong upper body muscles.

When she graduated from the program, Audrey left with a detailed record of her progress on the machines. She then took this record to the local group that managed her maintenance program so they could co-ordinate and carry on the work Audrey started at the hospital rehab program. She also left with a booklet illustrating the exercises she could do at home without machinery.

"But the most important thing I learned in this room was how to breathe properly," says Audrey. She learned both pursed-lip breathing and diaphragmatic breathing. "I was taught how to slow down my breathing, how to get control. The trick lies in breathing gently — not heaving breaths in and out. I learned to breathe in through my nose and then out — gently — through my mouth. No forcing. That really helped me with my walking." As she says this, Audrey is strolling into the gymnasium of the rehab centre.

"The first time I was in the gym, I walked one length and I was short of breath," she says. "By the end of the program, I was trotting back and forth, without feeling too bad. I was physically more fit, plus I could pace myself better and I wasn't afraid of breathlessness, since I knew how to control it. I was smarter about *how* I was walking. I'd stop if I needed it. Here's what I learned: 'Hold it, girl! Stop! Sit down!' Within five minutes, I'll be settled down. And then I'd carry on."

Audrey's rehab experience focused on increasing her levels of endurance, incorporating exercise into her life, improving her breathing, and learning to use her COPD medications better. Not everyone's experience will be identical. Audrey, for example, needed no help from the dietician — her weight was within the normal range, and she was eating a well-balanced diet. She and her husband had adapted their home and routines to her needs and therefore had no need for an occupational therapist. Mentally, both she and her family were coping well with the challenges of COPD, so there was no need for psychological counselling or help from the social worker.

Teamwork proved to be one of the greatest motivators for Audrey during her time in the program. "I started thinking about all the people who were helping me as my team. I didn't want to let them down, so I worked hard to do what they asked me." And the program delivered unexpected benefits: "My kids and my husband worry less about me now because they know I'm more independent, I can do more things for myself."

But rehab is not magic, Audrey advises. "Rehab will not work for you unless you want to do it and you have the urge to change. And you have to be committed to practising what you've learned after you leave the program. You go right downhill if you don't keep exercising. Rehab taught me that if I don't do these exercises, I'll go backwards. I'm not going to lie down and die. I'm stubborn. I carry on."

The Community-Based Rehabilitation or Maintenance Program

For every large, formal rehabilitation program in Canada, there are many smaller ones, like the Better Breathers Club that registered nurse Brenda Hannivan coordinates in the small Ontario town of Port Perry.

Brenda works for VitalAire Healthcare, an oxygen supply company. Her job takes her into the homes of people with lung disease. She discovered, to her dismay, that many of the people she was helping with oxygen therapy didn't know how to use their other medications very well. Puffers posed a real challenge for some. One of her patients actually emptied the contents of his puffer into a spoon and swallowed the medication. Others were leading completely sedentary lives, fearful of the breathlessness that might accompany exercise. Still others wanted to stop smoking but had no idea where to turn for guidance or support.

The nearest rehabilitation program was 60 km south of Port Perry in Oshawa, but most of Brenda's patients didn't even know the program existed. Their doctors had never discussed rehabilitation with them. In any case, it was too long a drive for many, particularly in the winter.

Brenda saw a need and decided — with help from others at the local hospital and The Lung Association — to fill it. She calls the Better Breathers Club an "educational support program." She began by advertising the program in the local newspaper and dropping off brochures in the hospital emergency department, doctors' offices, pharmacies, and local visiting nurses' offices. She sent letters to all the local doctors, telling them about the program and the proven benefits of pulmonary rehabilitation.

The program operates the third Wednesday of every month at Lakeridge Health, Port Perry's hospital. Brenda has a loyal group of nearly twenty regulars, most of whom have been with the program since its inception. Better Breathers caters to those with all types of chronic lung disease, including asthma, emphysema, and chronic bronchitis. Before a person can participate in the program, he or she must first be referred by a physician and seen by the hospital's physiotherapist, who reviews his or her condition to ascertain whether the patient can take part in the exercise component of the program.

The first half-hour of every session is devoted to group exercises led by a physiotherapist. The physiotherapist works on stretching, muscle strengthening, and breathing exercises. A casual class follows, often led by visiting speakers. Brenda sets a comfortable tone, serving juice and cookies, and encourages family members to attend. "We get patients bringing along their young grandchildren," she says. But despite the casual atmo-sphere, the topics discussed are serious, ranging from anatomy to nutrition to stress management to the importance of flu vaccinations to respite care and nursing homes. Brenda has even led a field trip to a pulmonary function lab, where patients learned about spirometry and had their FEV_1 checked. After the serious stuff, the participants might play a hand or two of euchre.

"We try to broaden everyone's horizons so they can make informed decisions on how to improve their lifestyle and know when to see a doctor," Brenda says. "We don't force them to do things. Motivation must come from the patients themselves. They have to want to exercise and eat right. We give the information and support they need."

Once people join Brenda's group, they tend to stick with it even though they may have heard the programs before. "They tell me they've forgotten the information," she says with a laugh. "But I know they've come for the camaraderie. This program helps them cope with a difficult disease."

To find out whether a program like this is offered in your community, contact your local hospital or The Lung Association in your area.

The Self-Directed, At-Home Rehabilitation Program

Many people with COPD achieve gratifying gains in the activities of daily living and their health working on their own. Bigger is not always better. It depends on the person, his or her physical and mental condition, and level of personal motivation.

Let's look at some practical ideas and guidance about tending your body — breathing, exercising, and eating right — that you can do on your own.

Breathing, exercising, and eating right, combined with the medications she uses for her COPD, have helped keep Audrey's disease under control these past few years. Although Audrey learned to tend her body at a formal pulmonary rehabilitation program, she's been applying much of what she learned on her own, keeping herself in excellent physical shape. She's also had help from a pulmonary exercise maintenance program she attends twice weekly.

Remember: before embarking on any breathing exercises or other exercise program, speak to your doctor, who will provide instructions or refer you to a professional who can help you.

Breathing Right

"I spent years grabbing for breath," says Audrey. "I'd be gasping — inhaling and exhaling rapidly through my mouth. And, instead of the deep breaths I wanted, I was only getting in small amounts of air. It made me completely exhausted and panicked. I know now that shortness of breath is not going to kill you. All you need to do is slow down your breathing. Keep it under control. The way you do that is by practising your breathing. Sounds crazy, learning how to breathe. We all do it naturally. But when you have COPD you need to do things a little differently."

Audrey's "grabbing for breath" was exhausting the breathing muscles of her abdomen, chest, and neck. A physiotherapist taught Audrey the breathing exercises outlined below. With regular practice, she's learned to control her breathing, adopting a slower, deeper breathing pattern. This, in turn, has allowed her to walk, talk, cook, shop, exercise, and drive without worrying about shortness of breath and fatigue.

DON'T PANIC — SOS BREATHING FOR SOB (SHORTNESS OF BREATH)

1. Stop and rest in a comfortable position.
2. Get your head down.
3. Get your shoulders down.
4. Breathe **in** through your mouth.
5. Blow **out** through your mouth.
6. Breathe in and blow out as fast as necessary.
7. Begin to blow out longer, but not forcibly. Use pursed lips if you find it effective.
8. Begin to slow your breathing.
9. Begin to use your nose.
10 Begin diaphragmatic breathing.
11. Stay in position for five minutes longer.

Remember: Breathlessness resulting from effort is uncomfortable but not in itself harmful or dangerous!

SOB Positions

1. Sitting — Your back against the back of the chair. Your head and shoulders rolled forward, relaxed downwards, hands and forearms resting on thighs, palms turned upwards. Do not lean on your hands! Feet on floor, knees rolled slightly outwards. Do SOS for SOB until breathing returns to normal.
2. Sitting — Leaning back into chair in a teenage slouch position, your head rolled forward, shoulders relaxed downward, hands resting gently on stomach, feet on floor, knees rolled outward. Do SOS for SOB until breathing returns to normal.
3. Sitting — Head and shoulders rolled forward, relaxed and down, table or chair in front of bed, arms folded, resting on pillow on table, feet on floor or stool, head on folded arms on pillow on table. Do SOS for SOB until breathing returns to normal. (This position may be used while standing, arms resting on kitchen counter or back of chair — not leaning! Knees bent slightly, one foot in front of the other.)
4. Standing — Leaning with back to wall, pole, etc. Feet slightly apart and a comfortable distance from the wall, head and shoulders relaxed. Do SOS for SOB until breathing returns to normal.

Reprinted with permission from The Lung Association's Breathe Easy — A Program about Living with Lung Disease.

BREATHING TIPS

Depending on the severity of your condition, some of the exercises we will describe may not be recommended for you. Speak to your doctor.

- Rest if you feel dizzy at any time during your breathing exercises.
- To perfect your technique, try practising without clothes in front of a mirror. Watch your chest, abdomen, neck, and mouth.
- Drink plenty of water just as you would during any type of exercise.
- Breathing exercises should be done in conjunction with your medications, not in lieu of them.
- Time your exercises for the part of the day when you feel most energetic.
- Take your bronchodilator inhaler several minutes before you exercise.
- Use oxygen during exercise if so advised by your doctor.

Pursed-Lip Breathing

Getting air out of your lungs is a problem when you have COPD. Because your airways tend to collapse, air becomes trapped in your lungs, hyper-inflating them and making it difficult for you to breathe in fresh air. Pursed-lip breathing is an effective way of getting some of that trapped, stale air out of your lungs and of slowing down your breathing. Exhaling using pursed-lip breathing slows your breathing rate down and increases the pressure in your airways, keeping them open longer than if you were breathing normally and thus allowing trapped air to leave the lungs.

Pursed-lip breathing is simple to do:

1. Inhale a normal amount of air through your nose. Keep your mouth closed and breathe in slowly.
2. Exhale slowly through your mouth. Keep your lips pursed, blowing out as if you're whistling slowly.
3. Try to exhale twice as long as you inhale. It can be helpful to count. Count to two when you inhale, count to four when you exhale.
4. If you practise pursed-lip breathing when you're relaxed, you'll find it becomes natural to do when you find yourself breathless or when

you're attempting activities that cause shortness of breath, such as walking or recovering from a stair climb.

Diaphragmatic Breathing

The diaphragm is the main breathing muscle. The hyperinflated lungs of the COPD patient tend to flatten this muscle. Once flattened, the diaphragm can't do its job of bringing fresh air into the lungs. But many COPD patients can learn to use this muscle more effectively. In fact, this can be a very relaxing exercise.

It might take some practice to master the technique for diaphragmatic breathing:

1. Sit in a comfortable chair. Relax your shoulders.
2. Place your hands lightly on your abdomen.
3. Breathe in slowly through your nose. You want to feel your abdomen rise out under your hands.
4. Breathe out through pursed lips. Your abdomen should fall inward.

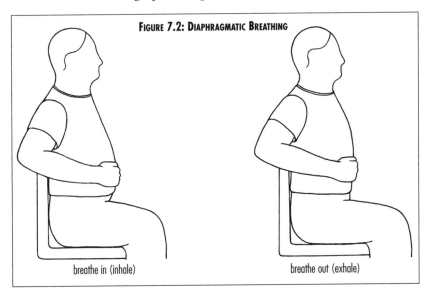

FIGURE 7.2: DIAPHRAGMATIC BREATHING

breathe in (inhale)   breathe out (exhale)

Chest Wall Breathing

The intercostal muscles located between your ribs are also important breathing muscles. To prevent these muscles from tightening, work on expanding and contracting them:

1. Relax your neck and shoulders.
2. Place your hands on your ribs.
3. Breathe in slowly through your nose. Feel your rib cage expand.
4. Breathe out through pursed lips. Your rib cage should contract.

Posture

Like your mother said, sit up straight! Notice we said "sit," not "stand"? If you have the choice, sitting is a good way to save your energy. Sit to peel potatoes, sit to brush your teeth, sit to dress, sit to dry the dishes, sit to water the flower beds, sit on a bath stool in the shower. But, sitting or standing, always maintain good posture. Hunched shoulders and poor posture don't allow your chest to expand to its full capacity, making it more tiring for you to breathe.

Relaxing your shoulders makes it easier to breathe. Sit with your hands palms up in your lap. When your hands are palms down on your knees, your shoulders tend to rise, which tenses up your shoulder and neck muscles.

Coughing Techniques

Some COPD patients, like Audrey, produce excessive amounts of mucus. This is common in patients whose COPD is dominated by chronic bronchitis. Those who suffer predominantly from emphysema often don't have a problem with too much mucus. For those who do, however, the trick lies in getting rid of it. Not only does excessive mucus make it harder to breathe but it's also a friendly environment for breeding lung infections.

"The trick is to avoid too much coughing," advises Audrey. "A hacking, retching cough is too hard on you, using up too much energy. Start by concentrating on your breathing. Slowly take a deep breath that comes from your midriff. Hold it for a second or two, then cough. That should bring some mucus from your lungs up into your throat. Cough again — like a cat getting rid of a hairball — and get a tissue ready. Once you've finished, try to avoid breathing in too deeply, otherwise you'll start a coughing fit. Stop for a bit and repeat the process, if necessary."

Audrey makes a point of clearing her lungs before she begins any of her exercise programs. "I find it makes my chest feel less tight," she explains.

Exercising Right

"Exercise, but know when to stop," says Audrey. Sounds like contradictory advice, but for a COPD patient it's precisely the way to get the most from your exercise.

When you're often short of breath, it's easy to slip into a lifestyle of inactivity. You feel lousy, you feel anxious. Will you be able to catch your next breath? Next to smoking, a pattern of inactivity is one of the worst things for a COPD patient. The longer you sit, the more out of condition your muscles become, the greater effort breathing requires, and, finally, the more short of breath you become. But you need to know when to stop exercising too. It's important to pace yourself so you don't find yourself uncomfortably breathless.

"It's easy to say we all need to exercise. Actually doing it is a lot tougher," chuckles Audrey. "I've organized my life so that exercising fits into it neatly. I've planned my exercise schedule in a way that's easy and pleasant to accomplish. After my workouts at the therapy centre, for example, we all go to Tim Hortons for some sustenance and then we play bridge afterwards. I make certain to do my stretching exercises every morning before breakfast and before I get off track doing other things."

Audrey's exercise regimen involves three elements:

— stretching exercises every morning,
— a daily walk, inside in the winter, outside in the summer, and
— one hour exercising on a treadmill and stationary bicycle, twice each week, at a therapy centre under the supervision of a respiratory therapist.

This program provides Audrey with three key types of exercise:

— **aerobic exercise** — By increasing the heart rate for a sustained period, aerobic exercise improves cardiovascular fitness, allowing your body to use oxygen more efficiently. Audrey's daily walks and twice-weekly workouts provide aerobic benefits. Swimming and cycling are other ways of obtaining this exercise.
— **resistance training** — Improving muscle strength and conditioning is important for COPD patients, who put extra demands on their breathing muscles. Audrey works on both her leg and arm muscles

JUST DO IT! EXERCISES YOU CAN DO AT HOME

Breathing is tough physical work for someone with COPD. To ensure you've got the energy and muscle power it takes to catch a breath — plus something left over to cope with daily living — it helps to be as physically fit as possible.

We know that exercise strengthens your hard-working respiratory muscles, allows your body to use oxygen more efficiently, and improves your overall strength and endurance. This makes exercise a cornerstone of the management of your COPD. And if you've already incorporated an exercise program into your life, you've made a decision you will never regret.

If you're thinking about exercising, there are a few things to learn:

1. See a doctor before beginning any exercise program. Ask whether you could benefit from using a walker or supplemental oxygen while exercising.
2. Use your bronchodilators **before** exercising, if appropriate.
3. Warm up **before** and cool down **after** exercising. This means **stretching** before all physical activity, including a simple walk. Not only is stretching relaxing, it improves your body's flexibility.

FIGURE 7.3: STRETCHING

Stretching by Bob Anderson (Shelter Publications) is a must-have sourcebook for stretches for all types of activity.

4. Include **aerobic exercise** — the type that works your heart and lungs — in your exercise regimen at least three to five times each week. It's best daily! Choose something you enjoy. Simple, inexpensive activities — like walking, swimming, stair climbing, riding a stationary bicycle — are all excellent aerobic exercises. (In winter, stroll in your local mall or use a stationary bicycle or treadmill — the investment is worth it.)

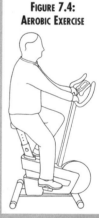

FIGURE 7.4:
AEROBIC EXERCISE

FIGURE 7.5:
RESISTANCE
TRAINING

5. Don't forget your muscles. **Resistance training** — working on your major muscle groups at least two days per week — is recommended for strengthening your body. Working with weights can be as easy as doing a series of elbow bends with a small soup tin in your hand. For some exercise ideas, check out *Living with COPD*, a publication of The Lung Association, available free in Canada by phoning 1-800-972-2636.
6. Remember to breathe and cough effectively and efficiently. Read about pursed-lip and diaphragmatic breathing in this chapter. Use it when you need it and practise it regularly.

> 7. Finally — and most important — make exercising fun. Do it with a friend. Listen to some great music while you stretch. Vary your activities. Experiment and find exercises you like. Listen to your body. Never exercise if you're in pain. Exercise when you're well rested. And set your own pace — it's not a race!

when pedalling a stationary bike that also has hand pedals. She finds strengthening her chest muscles has been particularly helpful for her breathing by making the muscles of her rib cage less tight.

— stretching — Audrey starts each morning with twenty to thirty minutes of stretching exercises. Part of the workout involves deep breathing, and loosening up chest, shoulder, and arm muscles.

Audrey is religious about her exercise routine, only opting out when she's feeling unwell. She's obviously found what's right for her, incorporating a variety of goodies into her routine. It didn't happen overnight. She spent time researching and pricing programs around town and ensuring that she'd be supervised properly. Audrey pays $50 a month for her biweekly sessions and is supervised at all times by a respiratory therapist. "It makes me feel more comfortable to have someone there who can take my blood pressure and blood oxygen levels," she explains.

Of course, not everyone would need this type of supervision and not everyone would want to be doing the things Audrey does. Like Audrey, you too can find the exercises that are right for you. Think about an aquafit course, or tai chi, or yoga. But be realistic. Will you really enjoy it? Do you need the company of others to encourage you? Have you taken into consideration any other health concerns that might impede your exercise program? You might need supplemental oxygen to exercise. Ask your doctor.

Don't be surprised if your doctor recommends plain old walking. It's simple, cheap, provides great aerobic exercise, and can be done anywhere, including your home, apartment hallway, or shopping mall. Audrey is a walking fan. Step into her kitchen and you'll see pairs of walking shoes lined up by her back door. "I walk all year long. In the winter, I walk in the house and on the treadmill at the therapy centre. In the summer, I walk around my neighbourhood. For my summer walks, I set a goal. Let's say

I want to be able to walk to the neighbourhood shopping centre. But I don't walk that far the first day I'm out, I work up to it. I always remember to stop when I feel I'm becoming breathless. That way I keep my shortness of breath under control. I know all my neighbours, so I can always go sit on someone's front steps if I get too short of breath. I also remember not to get too far from home. I need enough wind to retrace my steps back. On very hot, humid, or smoggy summer days, I stay indoors. If things are better by evening, I might go out before I go to bed. I've gotten into the habit of listening to the air quality reports on the radio and television. If the air quality is poor, I stay inside." And Audrey makes a point of warming up and cooling down before her exercise. She stretches before she sets out on her walk and slows her pace to cool down as she rounds the bend toward home.

You're probably thinking you could never keep up with Audrey. Bet you could. She moves slowly and surely. She never rushes. In fact, she often stops to catch her breath. She's no Hercules. What Audrey has that so many are missing is motivation. "I'm addicted to exercise," she explains. "I have to keep it up or else I lose ground. I'm so much more alert after I exercise. I'm able to breathe better. For me, the effects are immediate. That 'pluggy,' tight feeling leaves my chest. I just feel so much better and I can keep doing the things I love." Two of Audrey's grandchildren are getting married this summer and Audrey wants to attend every shower and party and both ceremonies. To do so, she's got to stay in shape, and that means walking, stretching, and pedalling!

Eating Right

Audrey is not a good example for this section of the chapter. Not because she doesn't eat well — she does. But food has never been a problem for her. She's currently at an ideal body weight. That's not always the case for COPD patients. Janet and Raymond are perfect examples of the two extremes. Maintaining a healthy weight is a constant battle for both of them. And both work diligently at winning the war. "It's simple," says Janet. "You don't eat properly, you get sick. And if I get a chest infection, I land in the hospital. Eating well keeps me healthy."

Janet is underweight. This is not an uncommon condition for COPD patients with predominantly emphysema. When you're fighting for every breath, you're using up to one and a half times more calories than someone without lung disease. Plus, eating — chewing in particular — can be tiring and cause shortness of breath. Like Janet, many COPDers find that filling up on food makes them feel breathless. Food becomes something to be avoided.

"You can't be too rich or too thin" the saying goes. In fact, you can be too thin when you have COPD. A poor diet can result in a lack of energy. No energy can mean no exercise, which leads to wasting muscles, which makes breathing even more difficult. When foods are avoided, you run the risk of missing out on vitamins and minerals essential to health. The result is an increased risk of infection and illness.

Raymond, on the other hand, is overweight. Obesity brings another set of problems to COPD. A big belly tends to place pressure on the diaphragm, pushing it up into the chest cavity. Not only is the diaphragm now unable to work efficiently, but it also limits the ability of the lungs to expand. Thus, the capacity of already damaged lungs is further reduced. Obesity also tends to place additional demands on the heart and lungs, which are already stressed by COPD. (An exercise program would be a good way for Raymond to lose a few pounds and improve his overall fitness level.)

Although their problems are different, Raymond and Janet are working to accomplish the same goal — a healthy, well-balanced diet. A copy of "Canada's Food Guide" is taped onto Raymond's refrigerator, and he consults it regularly when planning his meals. The food guide is a great starting point for all COPD patients. It provides information on the four food groups (grain products, vegetables and fruit, milk products, and meat and alternatives) and the number of servings you'll need from each group. Best of all, "Canada's Food Guide" is free of charge. You can request the guide from Health Canada, A.L. 0913A, Ottawa, Ontario, K1A 0K9. It's also available on the Health Canada Web site at www.hc-sc.gc.ca.

"Canada's Food Guide" is a starting point for COPD patients, but a few modifications are necessary to accommodate their special needs. Eating can be a struggle for Janet: "I really suffer if I eat a large meal — I feel as if I'm choking. I make sure that I go to restaurants where I can order a half-portion, and at home I eat several small meals during the day rather than three big ones." Janet makes sure to drink plenty of water throughout the day. She keeps her larder well supplied with food for those days when she's not feeling well enough to go out. And she buys foods that are easy to prepare — yogurt, fresh fruits, eggs, peanut butter, vegetables, and milk. She's always on the lookout for high-calorie, high-fat foods. Many people like Janet find that nutritional supplements like Ensure and Carnation Instant Breakfast are good ways to increase their caloric intake.

Raymond loves to cook and loves to eat. He knows he needs to stay away from fat-laden prepared foods like potato chips and baked goods. He also wants to avoid the high amounts of salt that many prepared and canned foods contain, knowing that too much salt can contribute to retention of fluid in the tissues. He works hard at preparing his own food.

EATING TIPS FOR COPD PATIENTS

Eat smaller meals. If you feel uncomfortable after eating a large meal, consider several snack-size meals during the day.

Time your meals. If you eat your main meal early in the day, you'll have energy to take you through your day.

Replenish your fluids. Drink six to eight glasses of liquid every day. Liquids should not contain caffeine. Fluids serve to thin the mucus in your lungs, making it easier to clear.

Increase fibre to avoid constipation. Straining to have a bowel movement requires energy and can leave you breathless. When you increase fibre intake, make sure you drink plenty of liquids.

Reduce the amount of salt in your diet. Too much salt can cause your body to retain fluid. Additional fluid in the tissues around the lungs and heart can contribute to breathing problems.

Make sure to get enough protein. Protein maintains and repairs the cells of the body. Milk is an excellent, easy source of protein.

Consider your medications. Some medications affect the way your body functions, making a change in your diet necessary. Diuretics, for example, cause your body to lose potassium, a mineral important for muscle function. In this case, you need to supplement your diet with potassium-rich foods, such as bananas, milk, and meat. Certain medications may make you feel ill or reduce your appetite. Ask your doctor or pharmacist whether there are ways of taking your medications that can minimize those side effects.

Avoid gas-producing foods. Consider using an antiflatulence product such as simethicone (Ovol 180). Many COPD patients suffer from excessive gas because of the air they swallow with their quick and laboured breathing (the technical term is **aerophagia**). Swallowed air tends to bloat the stomach and intestines, making breathing more laborious.

Supplement with vitamins and minerals. Vitamin and mineral supplements may be necessary, particularly for those who are malnourished. Speak to your doctor about what, if anything, you should consider taking.

Balance your diet. Remember "Canada's Food Guide" and be sure to select foods from the basic food groups each and every day.

Taped to his fridge you'll find a collection of wholesome soup recipes, and sitting in the freezer are small packages of homemade meals. Raymond will cook large batches of soup, for example, then freeze them in meal-size packages so he always has a healthy meal on hand if he feels the impulse to eat. Plus, if he's not feeling great, he simply warms up a prepared meal. "Living alone, cooking can be tough," he comments. "Sometimes you don't feel like cooking or eating. But it's dangerous for your health to slip into a routine of tea and toast or junk foods."

As with many COPD patients, lung disease is not Raymond's only health problem. He has diabetes and has an ileostomy (a portion of his bowel has been brought out to the abdominal wall where wastes are collected in a bag). Both place restrictions on his diet. To learn how to cope, he consulted a dietician as part of his pulmonary rehabilitation. (If you'd like to speak to a nutritionist, ask your doctor for a referral. Most hospitals have a dietician on staff.) The dietician taught Raymond how to read package labels and recipes and how to stock his fridge with foods that are good for him. He also belongs to a support group at his local Lung Association and he's found it a good source of dietary information. He scours the food section of the local newspaper for new recipes. And he's resigned himself to a constant battle with the bulge. "I love to eat," he says with a shrug.

Now that you've learned how to get your body back into shape, move on to chapter 8 for some practical tips on how to cope with the day-to-day challenges of living with COPD.

8

Living with COPD — Practical Tips for Making the Most of Your Life

*I*t's been said that the art of life is to know how to enjoy a little and endure much. Peg argues that if you strive to enjoy your life, you won't think so much about enduring it. "Once you've accepted the fact that COPD will change the way you live your life, then it's up to you to find ways to make your life better."

Peg's Story

"I don't want to sit around for the rest of my life but I can't run up three flights of stairs anymore, either. I've got a dilemma on my hands and I need to solve it so I can get on with my life." That's Peg, who, until she was diagnosed with COPD in 1992, had spent an active, outgoing life working, raising a flock of kids, skiing, taking courses, volunteering — you name it. Then she hit the brick wall of COPD head on. "My first inclination was to stay home," she recalls. "I didn't want anyone to see me short of breath and helpless. I was tired. I was mad. I refused to accept the diagnosis."

Peg slowly came to the realization that she'd stopped doing almost everything she'd once loved. She had allowed herself to become trapped by her COPD. She began reclaiming her life after a stay at a local rehabilitation program where she learned how to solve her dilemma and get on with her life. She's certainly not as physically active as she once was but she's back to being her extroverted self and is busy at home and active in her community.

Peg's story is not unusual for COPD patients. Worried about breathlessness and depressed by their diagnosis, people begin to avoid activities. Why go grocery shopping? Let someone else do it for you. Why go for a walk with a friend? They might see you gasping for breath.

This is how COPD traps you. Forsaking activities leads to an increasingly sedentary lifestyle. This, in turn, leads to an ever declining state of physical health characterized by more breathlessness and fatigue. Remember, breathing is an endurance sport, and you need to have your breathing muscles in good shape to compete. Allowing them to get out of shape by adopting a sedentary lifestyle makes breathing even more difficult. Your out-of-shape muscles need to work harder than ever to allow you to catch a breath. Before you know it, even the easiest activities make you breathless.

But there's more. As the song says, "you don't know what you've got till it's gone." The activities you've given up were what got you up and out of the house, made you proud of what you could accomplish, and kept you in contact with your friends and neighbours. Without them, life becomes pretty boring. Depression and anxiety can be common bedfellows of COPD.

How can you break out of the COPD trap? Not everyone's like gregarious Peg. Nor does everyone have the opportunity to attend a formal rehabilitation program. But, according to Peg, once you've made the decision to keep busy, it's a matter of basic common sense. "It's learning simple things. If I peel potatoes sitting down rather than standing up, I'll save energy. If I put 'em in a pot and cook 'em without peeling them, I'll save even more energy. If I can do it, anybody can." But first, you must be committed to change. "Change is what I do now," says Peg. "If you're willing to adopt a flexible attitude — and eat your potatoes unpeeled — you're well on the way." In other words, don't take on more than you can handle, and if you find yourself becoming tired or breathless, quit! You can always try again another day.

"Energy conservation" is what a physiotherapist would call this process. At the rehabilitation program, Peg learned the "Ps" of energy conservation: Pacing, setting Priorities, and Planning. "I'd add Patience to that list," she states, "because you need to be patient with yourself when you're learning how to change the way you do things."

Pacing has always been a problem for busy Peg. Finding the right balance is difficult for her because she always wants to go at full tilt. But she's learned she'll feel much better if she works at a slow, steady pace and remembers to take breaks. "I used to try to keep up with my daughter when we were walking through malls. I finally sat her down and told her that I cannot rush. I need to walk slowly and I may need to sit down periodically." She's learned that rushing is a good way to start a bout of breathlessness.

Peg has also learned to "just say no!" "I don't do anything I don't want to do," she explains. "And I've reduced my obligations accordingly." Peg gives the example of one of her volunteer activities. She completes income tax forms for seventy-five seniors in her community. "But I do it all at my convenience. Morning is the best time for me to work. I fade in the afternoon, so I only work on the forms before lunch. And if I don't feel like doing it, I stop. I don't want to get myself into a stressful situation."

Peg has figured out the most important things for her to accomplish each day, and that's what she tackles first. "Slow and steady wins the race," she says. She works slowly and takes breaks whenever needed. "I have my 'standing place' in the kitchen," she explains. "When I find I'm getting out of breath from talking or working, I stand at a counter where I have a collection of crossword puzzles. I find that by standing, leaning on the counter, and working a crossword puzzle, I can take my mind off my breathing and catch my breath without becoming panicked. Before you know it, I'm back to normal."

Priorities are important in your life, and COPD will change them. Setting priorities is a matter of figuring out what you want to do with your life and recognizing that you can no longer do as much as you once did. "You're not going to be able to do all of your ironing in one afternoon. You're not going to be able to keep up with your grandchildren on a bike ride. But there are other things you can do — it's up to you to find them," she explains. "The first thing is to accept the fact that things have changed. Next, start finding ways to make your life better."

"There are certain things I won't do," Peg says. She admits that she is still embarrassed about others seeing her breathless. She and her husband,

Harold, used to attend a series of concerts each year. But she felt her coughing was interrupting the performances. Just the thought of going to a concert stressed her out. They decided they didn't need to go to the concerts, they'd listen to CDs instead. Peg once loved digging in the dirt of her garden. She's now delegated the digging to Harold. But she still gardens in her own way, accompanying him to garden centres and supervising his work in the garden ("I think I prefer the rose bush over there!").

But politics is something that Peg refuses to give up. Deputy reeve of her township, she'll organize her entire day around attending an evening council meeting. And she continues to be devoted to her friends, staying connected through the phone. "It's so good for me to be able to phone a friend. If I'm not feeling great, I always have someone to phone who'll take my mind off my sickness. I've learned that I can't do everything myself. There are many times when I ask for help."

Planning is an easy task for the well-organized Peg. But, despite her skills, she's had to make some tough emotional decisions. Using a walker was the toughest. She wanted to keep travelling and shopping but was finding both tough. "A respiratory therapist at the rehabilitation program suggested that a walker would allow me to keep moving around. 'Me? A walker? I don't think so!' That was my first reaction. For me, using a walker was a sign of weakness, but I really wanted to keep moving. Now I think it's the best thing. I can sit on it when I'm tired and, when I'm shopping, I can use it to place my purse and purchases. I've used it for four years now and I use it anywhere and anytime I need to walk for any distance. It's great, and part of the cost was covered by government health insurance."

Peg has all sorts of practical planning tips:

- "I don't like to rush around the house," she says. "So I've organized things to be handy to me. For example, I have a cordless phone that I carry in my pocket. When the phone rings, I don't have the horrible feeling of missing the call because I can't run for the phone."
- "Whenever I go into a new place, I check it out to see where the bathrooms and benches are. That means I won't be in a panic to locate them later. And I never stand when I can sit."
- "I always have a good fat cushion with me. If I become breathless,

117

I lean on it in my lap, folding my arms on top of it, palms up. Then I do my pursed-lip breathing."

 Peg's kitchen is super-organized. It is tiny and everything is within easy reach. Items are stored in such a way that Peg doesn't have to lift her arms over her head to reach them.

Lorraine's Story

Lorraine's husband, Larry, is a pragmatic man. He and Lorraine have been in their home for thirty-seven years, and they don't want to move. Lorraine's mobility is restricted in two ways. Not only is she tethered to an oxygen unit but she's also easily fatigued by exertion. For the past few years, Larry and Lorraine have been tinkering around the house. Their goal? They both want Lorraine to continue enjoying her home and to

LORRAINE

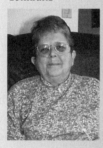

She is determined, intelligent, and she laughs all the time. It's easy to see why people like her, why people want to do things for her. Right now, in fact, a team of health care professionals in London, Ontario, is searching for a new lung for Lorraine. Because of the extensive damage done to her lungs by COPD, she is on the list to receive a lung transplant.

The first thing Lorraine does when you enter her sunny family room is haul out a photo album. "That's me last year at Myrtle Beach," she says, proudly pointing at a photo of a smiling woman on a golf course. "You can't see it, but I was hooked up to oxygen the entire eighteen holes." This woman is not in denial. She's not pretending she doesn't have a severe disease that's threatening her life. But for Lorraine and her husband, Larry, acceptance doesn't mean sitting around waiting for the end. "You've got to do what you've got to do," she says.

Family traditions are important in Lorraine's life. She and Larry, married for forty years, live in the house where they raised their two kids. They live just down the street from the house where Lorraine was born sixty years ago. Her daughter lives right across the street. Lorraine's two granddaughters are regular visitors. Everyone in her family smoked — father, mother, uncles, and aunts — cigarettes, cigars and pipes. "I started as a teenager," she recalls. "It was the natural thing to do in our family, and I didn't have the sense to do things differently."

In 1989, spurred by her doctor's warnings and concerned about her mother's health (she too had COPD), Lorraine convinced her mother that they should quit together. "If you quit, I can too," said Lorraine. "That was our deal." For the next five years, Lorraine never felt better. "Larry and I would travel south and we'd walk miles and miles on the beach."

She experienced her first bout of debilitating breathlessness in 1994. "I knew something was ensure that she'll be able to live as independently and actively as possible.

On the outside, Lorraine and Larry's bungalow looks like the rest of the tidy homes lining their street. Inside reveals a different picture. First, it's impeccably clean and tidy. Lorraine finds that dust aggravates her breathing, so one of the first things the couple did was to remove all the broadloom and replace it with easy to clean hardwood floors. They also made the difficult decision to give away their cat, whose dander was also an irritant for Lorraine.

Larry lists the other changes the couple have made:

 "We made it easy for Lorraine to get from the house to the car. She used to leave the house by the side door, where there are several steps. Now we've made an exit out the back with no stairs."

seriously wrong with my lungs. But I caught my breath and kept quiet about it. I didn't want to admit that I might be in the same boat as my mother." But Lorraine couldn't keep her condition a secret for long — after that first episode, she was plagued by breathlessness. Her family doctor prescribed a bronchodilator. By 1995, she was visiting a respirologist, who diagnosed her COPD.

From 1994 to 1997, she remained physically active. In fact, these were the years she learned to golf. By 1997, however, her health was on a downward slide. "During bad times, I'd be going four or five times every weekend to the emergency department to have my bronchodilator medication delivered by mask and nebulizer."

Lorraine's respirologist persuaded her to try oxygen. "I didn't want any part of it. I was certain that it would confine me to the house. One Monday morning, a man appeared at the house and told me he was here to assess me for oxygen. I was furious with my doctor for talking me into this. But he was right. I realize now that I was furious at the situation I'd created for myself. And I was so wrong about the oxygen. It freed me more than I could imagine. That's how I could still golf last year. The fellow who supplies the oxygen has been great. He taught us how we can travel and get around easily with it."

Later in 1997, Lorraine spent five weeks as an inpatient at Ottawa's pulmonary rehabilitation centre. "Being around others who were using oxygen made me so relaxed about it," she says.

Despite her diligent approach to her disease, Lorraine's condition continued to worsen. By 1998, her respirologist began talking to her about the possibility of a lung transplant. She and Larry made their decision immediately. "We're practical people. If something's wrong, you fix it. This is how I can be fixed."

The rightness of their decision was confirmed by Lorraine's brush with death in 1999. Suffering from a severe viral infection, she was unconscious for six days and spent two weeks on a ventilator in the intensive care unit. Since that time, she has been waiting — in her sunny family room — for the phone call telling her that a new lung is waiting and her life is about to change.

"When it was time to renovate the bathroom, we made it completely accessible for Lorraine," says Larry. The tub is gone, replaced by a shower stall level with the floor — Lorraine can walk into it easily. A permanent seat is installed in the corner of the shower stall so Lorraine can rest if she needs to. Handles line the shower stall, giving Lorraine support if necessary. All her bathing supplies — soap, face cloth, and shampoo — are within easy reach.

When the basement steps became insurmountable for Lorraine, the couple installed an apartment-sized washer and dryer in their former front-hall closet. "It's not what you'd expect at your front door, but it works for us," chuckles Larry.

When it came time to replace their car, the couple purchased a van that was much easier for Lorraine to get in and out of.

A table and a comfortable, firm chair are located right beside the kitchen so that Lorraine can sit and watch Larry preparing dinner, or can sit while she helps get meals ready.

The couple renovated an old sunroom on the back of their home, just steps from the kitchen. There, Lorraine can easily prepare her own food without worrying about the length of her oxygen tubing. "We wanted a comfortable place for Lorraine to work and relax. We've fitted it up with a stationary bicycle and treadmill for her to exercise. She loves to crochet and all her materials are here right beside her easy chair. The television is in the room along with her books and photo albums. Plus, this room is the sunniest and nicest in the house. It has everything she needs — all in one place."

When the couple built a new deck, they designed it so that Lorraine could walk straight out from the house, with no steps to climb down.

"This was strictly for Lorraine's pleasure," explains Larry. "I transplanted our perennial garden from the front of the house to the back where Lorraine can see and enjoy it from her sunroom."

Don't be daunted by what Lorraine and Larry have done. Remember, they've been working away on their home for more than five years. All these changes didn't happen overnight. "We've done a little bit here, a little bit there," says Larry. And don't be put off by the expense. Take the time and you'll find bargains. Larry points to Lorraine's state-of-the-art stationary bike and treadmill. "We knew Lorraine needed this equipment but we didn't want to pay full price, so we watched the classified ads in the newspaper until we found what we needed at a price we could afford."

A Day in the Life — Tips from People Living with COPD

From the moment you wake until you head back to bed, there are countless ways to make your life easier and more pleasurable. Remember what Peg said about pacing yourself — if you're tired or breathless, quit! There will always be another day to sweep the floor, change your sheets, shop for groceries, whatever.

We heard a few basic tips for living with COPD repeated by nearly all the members of our group:

- Take it easy — don't rush!
- Spend some time planning your day. If you're not having a good day, don't push yourself.
- Save your activities for that part of the day when you have the most energy.
- Delegate the chores and tasks you can't do.
- Wait a while after you've eaten. Launching into an activity while your body is digesting is a recipe for breathlessness.
- Time your activities around taking your medication. You'll probably feel best right after you've taken your meds.
- Breathe! Don't forget to use your pursed-lip breathing.
- Sit! Take a breather if you need to. And don't stand when you can sit.

TEN TIPS TO EASE THE BURDEN OF COPD

1. **Getting Out of Bed.** Sleep in if you need to. If you don't have a clock to punch and you wake up feeling lousy, sleep in! But try not to make a habit of this. It's all too easy to slip into a sedentary lifestyle. Start your day with some stretching exercises. You can do some of them

in bed, if you'd like. Your bed should be easy to make. Pulling up a sheet and electric blanket will be far easier on you than making a bed with several quilts and comforters.

As well, organize your clothes the night before so you don't have to go searching for things in the morning. Dress sitting down on the edge of your bed or on a chair in your bedroom. Keep things you'll need in easy reach. Leave your shoes sitting beside your bed, for example, rather than down the hallway by the front door.

2. **Taking a Bath or Shower.** Remember the important principle: never stand when you can sit. Consider purchasing a bath stool for your tub or shower stall. You also might think about attaching a hand spray unit to your shower head. Grab bars in the shower can make standing up and getting in and out of the tub easier. Before you start your bath, ensure that you've got everything close at hand — soap, towel, shampoo. Wrapping yourself in a fluffy terrycloth robe can

---

HEALTHY BREATHING — INSIDE AND OUT
The Outdoor World
Air Pollution: "Health Canada Suggests 5,000 People a Year Die Prematurely Due to Smog," blares a 2000 newspaper headline. According to the Ontario Medical Association, the majority of illnesses attributable to smog can be traced to one of its major ingredients, fine particulate matter. When this poisonous matter is inhaled deep into your lungs it can further irritate your already inflamed airways and lead to a COPD flare-up.

What can you do to avoid "bad air"? If you happen to live in an area that is prone to smog conditions, the simplest and most effective way to avoid bad air is to stay inside during a smog alert. Listen to the radio, watch the television, and read the newspapers. When they warn of poor air quality and possible health risks, stay indoors, close your windows, and turn on your air conditioner. If you must go out during a smog alert, plan your errands to minimize the time spent outside a controlled environment (the car, an air-conditioned shopping mall, etc.). If walking around outside is unavoidable, you may want to consider wearing a mask over your mouth and nose to filter out the fine particulates in smog. Your local Lung Association has a selection of such masks for sale.

Other tips to help you avoid bad air include avoiding travel in rush hour along busy expressways. Also, think about taking your vacation in a rural location rather than a large urban setting.

If, in addition to your COPD, you also have allergies or asthma, avoid your triggers. You probably already know what they are. If you're allergic to cats, stay away from them. (Even a short visit can be harmful.) If it's dust, stay off dirt roads in the summertime. You get the idea!

Weather: Some like it hot, some like it cold! Arthur loves warm summer days but dreads the cold winter wind because he can't catch his breath. Jean doesn't have a big breathing problem in winter, but

---

do much of the drying you'd otherwise have to do with a towel. Remember to rinse out the tub after your bath. That way you won't have to clean it as often. Take your bath when you feel up to it. If you're feeling crummy in the morning, have your bath before bed or save it until the next day. Consider taking a "bird bath." A sponge bath using a basin and washcloth may be all you need some days and is much easier than a full-scale dunking.

3. **Putting Yourself Together.** Again, don't stand if you can sit. When brushing your teeth and hair, shaving, or applying makeup, sit if you need to. Use roll-on or solid deodorants rather than aerosols or sprays to avoid inhaling something that may be bad for your lungs. Similarly, avoid heavily scented or perfumed products. Most deodorants and hair products now come in unscented varieties.

    As for clothing, keep it loose! Get rid of tight bras and girdles, restrictive neckties, belts that bind. Avoid restricting your ability to

---

the heat makes her breathless, so in the hot and humid summer she hunts out air-conditioned places. When travelling, she'll call ahead to ensure that her lodgings are air-conditioned.

To catch his breath in the winter, Arthur bundles up well. He always wears a scarf that he wraps around his neck and over his mouth. "That way I can keep some warm air coming into my lungs," he explains. (Protective cold air masks are also available from The Lung Association.) He's careful to park his car as close as possible to where he's headed. And if he's walking outside in the winter, he always carries a cellphone. If the winter wind prevents him from hiking home, he'll call his wife or friends for a lift. Plus, he's invested in an automatic car starter so he always drives off in a toasty warm car.

The Inside World
Air Pollution: Those annoying drafts blowing through your house are probably good for you. Newer homes and condominiums, with their energy-efficient construction, cut down on energy costs but they also retain stale air that contains hazardous home pollutants. And there are plenty of things around the home that qualify as pollutants, ranging from tobacco smoke to the dustballs accumulating under your bed to mould and fungi growing in your basement.

If you have allergies and asthma in addition to your COPD, the best advice is also the simplest. Keep your triggers out of your home. Look at Lorraine's experience. She gave away her cat. Her home is impeccably clean and dust free. Her husband, Larry, is a fiend with the vacuum cleaner. Her floors are bare of carpets. No one is allowed to smoke in the house or wear perfumes or hair sprays.

Don't count on your furnace filter to keep the air in your home clean. That filter is designed only to keep dirt from entering the furnace. If you have a humidifier, keep it clean. A dirty humidifier can be a source of airborne mould and fungi. Similarly, ensure that gas stoves, water heaters, furnaces, and dryers are properly ventilated and wood stoves are airtight.

breathe easily. The looser your clothing around your neck, chest, and abdomen, the better. Women should think about wearing jumpers rather than skirts with tight waistbands. Instead of wriggling into tight pantyhose, what about pants and ankle socks? What about a cotton camisole rather than a tight bra? Men should think about suspenders rather than a belt. Both sexes can wear slip-on shoes rather than ones that tie up.

Make dressing easy. Avoid garments with fussy buttons and fasteners. It's far easier to put on something that does up in front. Consider using a long-handled shoehorn to put on your shoes so you won't have to bend over.

4. **Housework**. First and foremost, you don't have to do everything at once. Dividing chores into small, manageable bits is a great way of keeping on top of your housework. Here's where planning and organizing can really pay off.

Organize your work spaces in the house so the things you use most often are within easy reach. The kitchen is a good example. If you're a tea drinker, keep all your tea necessities together in one corner of your kitchen. Organize your refrigerator so the foods you use most are within easy reach. Consider getting a cart on casters that you can wheel around your home. This will eliminate the need for you to lift and carry heavy items — you can just push them along. You might consider equipping your cart with a long-handled reacher, like a set of tongs, for picking things off the floor or reaching a high shelf. When lifting, use your pursed-lip breathing. If you're carrying something heavy up the stairs and you find yourself becoming breathless, put it down and come back for it later.

Take care with cleaning products. Avoid using aerosols and sprays. Always work in a well-ventilated area when using any clean-

DO YOU NEED AN AIR CLEANER?

The discussion of clean indoor air might make you think you need an air cleaner. You've probably heard of HEPA (high-efficiency particulate air) filters, electronic air cleaners, and ion and ozone generators. Although some of these filters have been shown to remove particulate matter from the air quite effectively, the health benefits haven't been proven. It's felt that many of the particles that bother us are too small to be filtered out by these machines. The best way to keep your air clean is simply to keep your home clean.

ing product. Wear a mask when using these products and when dusting. To avoid kicking up excessive quantities of dust, consider using a slightly damp dust rag. Use a long-handled dustpan to avoid bending over.

5. **In the Kitchen.** Good nutrition is extremely important for people with COPD, and making things as easy as possible for yourself in the kitchen is a good first step to ensuring that you eat well. When you're feeling good, prepare extra food and freeze it in meal-size portions for those days when you're feeling lousy. Keep convenience foods on hand for those days when you don't feel great. A microwave oven can be a big help on this score. Always keep plenty of liquids on hand. Once again, don't stand when you can sit. Organize your kitchen so you can do as many tasks as possible while sitting down.

Not everything needs to be done at once. You can finish your meal and relax for a bit before you tackle the dishes, for example. Consider how you store your kitchen tools. If you always use one pot for cooking, do you need to put it away in a cupboard under the counter? Why not wash it and leave it on a burner on the stove? That will save you a few steps and the energy required to bend over to put it away and get it out for your next meal. It's all a matter of thinking things through and figuring out what's right for you.

6. **Getting Out and About**. You'll find detailed tips about travelling in chapter 12, but here are a few things to consider when you're getting around your own town. Plan ahead. If you haven't visited the place before, you can always phone ahead to see if you can get around. If stairs are a struggle for you, for example, you might want to find out whether you'll have to climb any.

Try to avoid travelling in rush hour. Not only can it be frustratingly slow, but the air quality is often bad. Keep an emergency kit in your car. Consider a cellphone. Think about obtaining a handicapped permit for your car.

7. **Shopping and Eating Out.** Shop in stores that make it easy for you. Some stores have staff to help you load groceries into your car, for example. A small store, organized efficiently, might save you steps. Make shopping easy for yourself. Don't shop when the crowds are out in force. Avoid the weekends and evenings. Think about using

the services of a mail-order company. You can buy everything from food to clothing through the mail, over the phone, or on the Internet these days. If trying on clothing in a small fitting room is daunting, make sure you can return items, then take them home to try on at your leisure.

If you're going to a restaurant, make certain it's not smoky. If you can't manage to eat large meals, go to a restaurant where you can order half-portions, or ask to take your leftovers home for an easy second meal.

8. **Keeping in Touch.** There are plenty of aids that will keep you in touch. Some people with COPD use a baby monitor to speak to their partners without having to shout or rush through the house. Others use walkie-talkies with longer ranges. If you spend time alone, you might consider using a personal help button, a home monitoring service that allows people to summon help when they need it. The panic button is worn around the neck or on the wrist and is pressed when help is needed. These buttons can be arranged through most home security companies.

9. **Back to Bed.** A cozy bed is a tempting place after a long day. But don't get into bed exhausted. If you take your time preparing for bed, you won't be breathless by the time you get there. Change into your pyjamas slowly. Ensure that you have everything you need set up on your bedside table long before bedtime. A phone (for emergencies) is a good item to have close at hand. But you'll also want some water, any medications you might need during the night, tissues, a night light (particularly if you need to get up during the night), a good book or remote control for your TV (for those sleepless nights).

You might consider finishing the day as you started it — with some exercises. This time, though, you'll want to relax your muscles. A good way of doing this is by concentrating on slow pursed-lip breathing. Make sure you're comfortable, then begin concentrating on relaxing each part of your body in turn. Tell yourself, for example, that your arms are heavy, warm, and relaxed. Then allow them to feel that way. Next, work on your legs. After several minutes, when you've finished your relaxation process, stretch your body long, with your arms over your head.

10. **The Pleasures of Life.** Stay connected! Loneliness and boredom can set in very quickly if you don't keep up with your friends and make some new ones along the way. Plus, having someone you can contact is a great support if you ever need help. The telephone is your best tool. Like Regis says, "Phone a friend."

Don't be afraid to reach out to new friends and neighbours. COPD support and seniors groups are a great way to meet new people. Taking up new activities can also open new doors. Not only will you meet new people but you'll feel enriched by learning something new, or just renewing your acquaintance with something you once loved. Look at the members of our group. They do everything from antiquing, to photography, to travelling, to golfing, to participating in municipal politics, to reading, to acquiring computer skills, to knitting, to walking, to birdwatching, to surfing the Internet. It's a matter of figuring out what your passion is and following it.

Where can you get other practical ideas? Consider joining a support group. The Lung Association is a good place to start looking for one. There you'll meet plenty of other people who are tackling the same issues.

9

"It's Never Too Late to Butt Out!" — A Smoke-Free Future

"Stop smoking!" How many times have you heard those words? If you have COPD and you're currently a smoker, aren't you tempted to smack the next guy who says that to you?

"Keep trying to quit." Don told us these were the most helpful words he received during his many attempts at quitting. "It's easy to tell someone to stop smoking, but it's so hard to stop," says Don. "If someone tells you to keep trying, it acknowledges the fact that you'll face setbacks. You might have to try a few times before you get it right. Quitting is probably one of the most difficult things you'll do in your life, and every smoker has to find his or her way out of the smoking addiction."

The decision to quit smoking is yours to make; no one else can make it for you. If you have COPD or think you may have the disease and you're still a smoker, reading this chapter is a big step for you. Many people with COPD don't report their symptoms to their doctors because they know there'll be pressure to give up the weed — and they feel they can't or don't want to. If this is you, please keep reading and keep trying. A key element of managing COPD is the prevention of further lung damage. And so far, the only way we know to accomplish that is to quit smoking.

Your FEV_1 can tell an interesting tale about both smoking and stopping. You may remember that your FEV_1 is an index of your lung function — as we age, our lungs age along with us. For healthy non-smokers, the age-related decline in FEV_1 is small — about 20 mL per year. But if you smoke regularly, your lung function could deteriorate up to four times faster than normal. The faster your lung function falls off, the faster you will reach a level of lung function low enough to make you feel rotten, with breathlessness and limitations to your activities. And the faster you will run out of lung power altogether and die. If you can stop smoking, usually your age-related decline in lung function will slow down and approach the natural age-related decline of non-smokers. So, it stands to reason, the sooner you quit smoking (say at age forty-five rather than sixty-five), the less likely you are to become disabled from your lung disease. If you stop early enough, you may never develop significant lung disability, and you will live longer too.

What We Know about Cigarettes

Nicotine, a drug as addictive as heroin or cocaine, physically addicts you to cigarettes. Via the cigarette, nicotine is absorbed through the lungs and hits the brain in a mere ten to nineteen seconds. That's faster than an injection can deliver the drug to the brain. The cigarette is a slick and efficient delivery system. Nicotine is not the toxin that causes COPD, cancer, or heart disease, however. Some four thousand compounds (including arsenic, nickel, formaldehyde, ammonia, and vinyl chloride) make up tobacco and tobacco smoke. These toxins are responsible for the diseases — respiratory disorders like COPD, and cancer and heart disease — that kill. Remember, it is the delivery system (the cigarette), not the drug (nicotine), that is responsible for the vast majority of tobacco-related disease.

Approximately 40,000 Canadians died in 2000 because of smoking. That's three times more than were killed by car accidents, murder, alcohol, AIDS, illicit drugs, and suicide combined! Tobacco is responsible for approximately one in five deaths in Canada, cutting more than fifteen years off the average smoker's life expectancy and killing about half of all long-term smokers.

These are astonishing statistics, but not surprising when you consider how many Canadians smoke. About 30 percent of all adult Canadians smoke, and the vast majority (86 percent) smoke daily. So what's the attraction? Nicotine usually gets the blame, but cigarettes are not only physically addicting, they hook smokers on a psychological level too. Smoking is an insidious habit. You smoke with friends on coffee break, you smoke when you're reading, you smoke when you're driving. Before you know it, you need cigarettes to enjoy the good times and to get through tough times and stressful social situations. Smoking becomes an integral part of who you are.

This combination of physical and psychological addiction makes it fiercely hard to kick the habit and nearly impossible to do without sources of help. No magic bullets exist to make the task easy. The average person will make three to four attempts to quit. Your doctor or The Lung Association can direct you to group smoking cessation programs. If you're interested in a program involving hypnosis, ensure that the leader is a professional properly trained in the field. If the program promises a one-session cure, run the other way. Acupuncture is also advertised as a way

DON

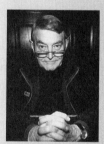

"I ate and slept my business," Don says. "I worked hard and I became financially independent at forty-five. I was smoking forty to fifty cigarettes a day back then. That's not hard to do when you're working till ten o'clock every night and you're under plenty of stress. And I wouldn't be here now talking to you if it weren't for those damn cigarettes."

Don trained as a civil engineer and opened his own business, designing and erecting steel buildings. His work took him all over Canada, from Vancouver to the Arctic Circle. His home life was busy too. He and his wife, Dolly, had seven kids in ten years. But he always found time to indulge his two passions: duck hunting and fishing. Lots of activity and lots of stress.

During childhood, Don suffered from recurring lung problems. His mother nursed him through several bouts of pneumonia. His health improved when he was a young man. And that's when he started to smoke. "I thought I was a big smart-ass. Everyone smoked in those days." Cigarettes quickly became an integral part of his stress-filled workdays. "It was the pressure. I had to light a smoke when I heard the phone ring. Just to get myself mentally prepared."

Around 1985, Don started to get recurrent lung infections during the winters. "As soon as I'd get a cold, it'd go right to the lungs. It was as if I had repetitive pneumonia. Early on, my family doctor told me to get rid of the damn cigarettes. I couldn't. My brain wanted that smoke." But it wasn't until he started spitting phlegm that he knew something was wrong.

Don was diagnosed with chronic bronchitis in 1997. At that time, his respirologist told him that he to stop smoking. Again, check out the credentials of the acupuncturist. Keep in mind that all these programs work best when combined with other supports.

Don't fall for "light" or "low-tar" cigarettes as an alternative to smoking cessation. Yes, these cigarettes may have less tar and nicotine than regular cigarettes, but many smokers make up for this decrease by changing the way they smoke — inhaling more deeply, for example. This makes these "light" cigarettes as "heavy" and harmful as regular ones.

Physically, nicotine exerts an addictive pull as strong as heroin. And cigarettes command a psychological hold on smokers that can be equally difficult to break. But people and medications can help you kick the habit once you've made the decision to quit. Attempts to quit that are most likely to succeed are those where the quitter starts out with as many supports as possible. Those supports can be personal — family, friends, doctors, co-workers, support groups — and medical — nicotine replacements (including the nicotine patch and gum), and bupropion hydro-

---

had approximately 70 percent of the lung capacity of a healthy person his age. And, pulling no punches, he told Don that if he wanted to shorten his life, then he should keep right on smoking. This was just the intellectual motivation Don needed — fear. And for now fear continues to keep him away from cigarettes. "I don't want to end my life on a breathing apparatus."

At seventy, Don has slowed down a bit. He's out of the steel building business and spends his time speculating in real estate and building houses now and again. He's still fishing and hunting, but he takes along someone younger to set the decoys and carry the outboard motor. "I know exactly how many steps there are to my boat dock — thirty-five. And they're getting tougher, especially if I'm carrying a can of gas, a case of beer, or my fishing tackle." He's particularly bothered by his diminishing abilities in comparison to others: "It peeves me right off to try to catch up to my wife when we're out walking."

Don approaches his COPD like the business person he is. He's established a goal and he'll do everything he needs to achieve it. He's not happy about having COPD. In fact, he's downright angry about it. But that diagnosis is what he's got to work with. He desperately wants to stay active, to keep up with his wife, to build more houses. Don has learned the signals and listens to them. It's all about keeping healthy and learning from your mistakes.

He tells the story about duck hunting in Manitoba last year. "We were getting up pre-dawn, pulling on clothes and setting out decoys. It was cold and wet. The prairie gumbo — a thick, clinging mud — made your boots weigh fifty pounds each. I sensed that I was going to get sick. But I didn't listen and I kept on going. Of course, I got a bad cold that went right to my chest. That was a lesson. I got the signal but I didn't listen. Next time, I'll pay attention."

chloride, a pill that may work on an "addiction centre" in the brain. People who quit cold turkey and with no supports in place tend to have significantly higher failure rates than those who seek out help and use other cessation strategies. Relapses are common. It typically takes three to four attempts before the quitting is permanent.

YOUR FEV₁ TELLS A STORY — THE RELATIONSHIP BETWEEN SMOKING AND LUNG FUNCTION

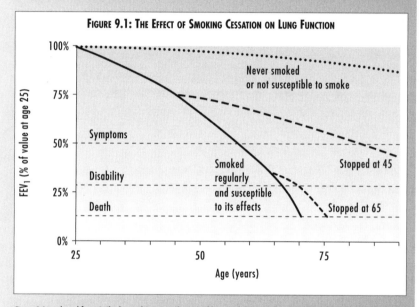

FIGURE 9.1: THE EFFECT OF SMOKING CESSATION ON LUNG FUNCTION

Figure 9.1 is adapted from C. Fletcher and R. Peto, "The natural history of chronic airflow obstruction," *British Medical Journal* 1977; 1: 1,645–48. Note: The line indicating the level of FEV₁ causing symptoms (e.g., breathlessness) is not fixed and will vary from person to person.

Figure 9.1 dramatically illustrates the effects of both aging and smoking on the functioning of our lungs as measured by FEV₁. In healthy non-smokers or smokers who are not affected by cigarette smoke, FEV₁ declines only minimally with age. In fact, the lung function of a seventy-five-year-old non-smoker is fairly close to that of a twenty-five-year-old! In smokers susceptible to the ravages of tobacco smoke, FEV₁ declines rapidly with age, reaching levels low enough to cause significant symptoms and disability in middle life. When smoking is stopped, however, the decline in FEV₁ slows down. If smoking cessation occurs early enough, COPD may not advance to significant symptoms, disability may be avoided, and early death may not occur.

Figure 9.2 reinforces the message that it's never too late to butt out. As you can see, the lower the predicted FEV_1, the lower the chances for surviving for the long term. Since stopping smoking can significantly reduce the decline in your FEV_1, it should make you think about stopping cigarettes earlier rather than later. And, as the chart shows us, even stopping at age sixty-five can make a big difference!

FIGURE 9.2: THREE-YEAR SURVIVAL IN COPD

FEV_1 % Predicted	% Surviving for 3 Years
> 50	~ 85
40–49	~ 82
30–39	~ 73
< 30	~ 60

Figure 9.2 is adapted from N.R. Anthonisen, E.C. Wright, and J.E. Hodgkin, "Prognosis in chronic obstructive pulmonary disease," *American Review of Respiratory Disease* 1986; 133: 14–20.

Second-Hand Smoking

As much as we think we are our own worst enemies, this isn't always the whole story. Make no mistake, the single biggest risk factor for the development of COPD, lung cancer, and heart disease is cigarette smoking. However, there is growing evidence that non-smokers who are exposed to other people's cigarette smoke over a long time are at risk for the same diseases that personal smoking causes. This is called second-hand or passive smoking, and is another reason why we should all work hard at smoking prevention.

Second-hand smoke exposure is linked to lung health problems especially in children and is one reason (the other is genetic) why COPD sometimes seems to run in families. Non-smokers inhale the carcinogens in nearby tobacco smoke, so it's not surprising that lung cancer is also related to passive smoking, especially in women. The excess risk of lung cancer in non-smoking women married to a smoker has been measured as between 15 and 24 percent.

It does not appear, however, that there is any excess cancer risk from exposure to environmental tobacco smoke (another name for second-hand smoke) in the workplace, in childhood, or during social activities.

How We Did It

To help you keep trying, Don, Mychelle, and Jean will tell you how they fought and won their battles against tobacco. They'll tell you what worked and didn't work for them — their setbacks, their supports, their tricks, their motivations, and, ultimately, their hard-won triumphs. You'll see that each of their stories is unique — what worked for some backfired for others. But there are many common themes in their stories.

Anyone who has tried to quit, or helped someone try, knows there's no quick fix. Gimmicks, lectures, threats, and scare tactics don't work. Interestingly, nearly everyone who's stopped goes through the same stages leading up to the actual "quit":

1. **No interest in quitting.** You're a smoker, you like it, and you're going to keep doing it.
2. **Thinking about quitting.** You start paying attention to things you hear about the dangers of smoking and start analyzing what your life would be like without the weed.
3. **Taking steps to stop.** You might contact The Lung Association, for example, for smoking cessation pamphlets or head to the bookstore for how-to books (more on that later). You line up supports — maybe you speak to your doctor about medical options. You decide on a "stop date."
4. **Quitting.** You figure out how you'll manage the first day, the first week, the first month without cigarettes.
5. **Staying on track.** You've quit. Now the challenge is to become, once and for all, a non-smoker.

Let's see how our group navigated those steps.

Don's Story

About fifty years ago, when I was still a teenager, my dad told me he quit smoking because he felt it was bad for his health. He asked me why I didn't quit. I couldn't give him an answer. I know now that I didn't want to quit. I enjoyed puffing on the weed and I didn't have the guts to stop.

A couple of months ago, I was talking to my son, Matthew. He's given up smoking for the second time. This time, he's using bupropion and it's working for him. We were trying to figure out why cigarettes have such a hold on us. "It's a reward," he told me. "You come in from doing a job outside, like cutting the grass, and you light up. You sit down with a good book after dinner, and you light up." He's right. For me, smoking was a pleasurable habit, a present I gave to myself.

After fifteen months off the weed, I'll still reach in my pocket, looking for my cigarettes. I'm still not out of it. I'll tell you, I want to smoke right now. Who the hell says I'll stay off the stuff now? But why would I want to do that? My body might want a cigarette but my mind says "no." I'm going to keep up the effort. I've decided that I don't want to end up on oxygen. I'm working at stabilizing my COPD and the only way I can do that is to stay off the weed.

I've learned a few things since I started trying to quit five years ago. I've had about three and a half quits since then. This has been my longest. The second longest lasted sixteen weeks. I thought I could start smoking again and hold it to only five cigarettes a day. Before I knew it, I was up to fifteen a day and then back to forty.

I've finally had the guts to hang on this time. So what's different for me this time? I was surprised the first couple of times I tried quitting how completely lousy I felt when I stopped smoking. I felt better when I was smoking. That was one of the reasons I'd start up again. Then I'd tell my wife, "Hey, I don't want to live to be a hundred anyway." She'd say, "The way you're going, you're not going to get anywhere near a hundred." After my second quit, I came to realize that, for me, quitting was purely an intellectual exercise. I had to convince myself that quitting was a good thing for me. And I had to recognize that my body was going to fight me all the way, pulling me back to the weed.

When I made it known that I'd firmly decided that I was going to quit, I had good support. My family and friends were encouraging. Two years ago, my respirologist gave me the intellectual motivation I needed. We had a good long talk about smoking. He didn't threaten or berate me but he was straight with me. He told me that stopping was the best thing I could do to prevent further damage to my lungs. And he told me that I had about 70 percent of the lung capacity of a healthy person my age. If I stopped smoking now, I had a good chance of stabilizing at that level rather than reducing it further. Fear motivated me. I was afraid that I would end up on a breathing apparatus.

WHERE TO GET MORE INFORMATION ABOUT QUITTING

More help is always better than less — particularly when you're trying to stop smoking. And there are plenty of sources of helpful tips and information available, much of it free!

Canadian Cancer Society

"One Step at a Time" is a self-help program for smokers and people helping others to quit. The program, based on the stages of the quitting process, includes three booklets: "For Smokers Who Don't Want to Quit," "For Smokers Who Do Want to Quit," and "If You Want to Help a Smoker Quit." These well-organized and informative booklets are free of charge. For copies contact the Cancer Information Service, toll-free at 1-888-939-3333; visit your local office of the Canadian Cancer Society; or go to the Cancer Society's Web site at www.cancer.ca/tobacco. The Cancer Society also has a smoker's helpline at 1-877-513-5333.

The Lung Association

"Get on Track: A Guide to Help You Quit Smoking" offers advice on how to get ready to quit, what to do when you're quitting, and how to stay a non-smoker after you've quit. The booklet costs $5.30 (Cdn.). The Lung Association also provides, free of charge, several short but informative pamphlets about a variety of topics, including cigarette smoking, nicotine addiction, drugs to help you quit, and second-hand smoke. For copies and information about these pamphlets, phone The Lung Association toll-free at 1-888-566-LUNG (5864), or go to their Web site at www.lung.ca.

The American Lung Association

7 Steps to a Smoke-Free Life is a book based on the American Lung Association's "Freedom from Smoking" program. This self-help book, written by Edwin B. Fisher, provides a complete overview of all the current stop-smoking strategies. The American Lung Association also has an excellent Web site with several articles on smoking cessation: www.lungusa.org.

Ontario Medical Association

A comprehensive review of the myths and facts of stop-smoking medications can be found at the OMA Web site: www.oma.org/phealth/stopsmoke.htm.

The National Jewish Medical and Research Center

The National Jewish Medical and Research Center, in Denver, Colorado, has helpful articles concerning lung diseases and smoking on its Web site, including "I Want to Stop Smoking (or Chewing) Tobacco." Visit www.njc.org.

Your Local Health Department

Local health departments often offer cessation and education resources for smokers who want to quit. Consult the Blue Pages of your telephone directory.

My doctor prescribed the nicotine patch for me. I know it works for a lot of people but the patch was not for me. I couldn't sleep with it on. If I didn't get the damn thing off before dinner, I'd have a terrible night with my mind working away at a thousand miles an hour. In the end, cold turkey worked for me. I woke up one morning and told myself: "I'm not going to smoke today." I've been repeating that sentence every day for the past fifteen months. I went clean and I've been squeaky clean for a long time. This time I've done things that have made it easy for me.

The hardest cigarette for me to give up was the first cigarette of the day, which I'd always smoked together with a cup of coffee. Now, my wife and I start our mornings with tea. And I went off beer for a while. A bottle of beer and a cigarette — they've gone together for me forever.

Giving up cigarettes has been the toughest thing I've ever done. It took me years to work up to it and it was totally mind over matter. I wish I could tell my dad that I had the courage to quit.

DON'S FIVE TIPS

Before you quit, spend some time assessing your habit. Where and when do you smoke? If you know the patterns of your habit, it's easier to break them. The most important cigarette to me was my first of the day, which I always had with a cup of coffee. I started to drink tea, and that made giving up that cigarette that much easier.

Stay away from places where there's smoking. I make an effort to go to smoke-free restaurants and coffee shops. No temptation.

Find something to do that takes your mind off smoking. I've started taking watercolour and computer courses. And I always keep toothpicks in my pocket to chew on.

Keep your life smoke-free. Don't allow smoking in your car, for example.

Take it one day at a time. Remind yourself every morning: "I'm a non-smoker!"

Jean's Story

To this day, I am enormously pleased with myself for quitting. My mother, who suffered from emphysema, never gave up smoking. She thought there wasn't much hope for her and she smoked to the end. I watched her die. And it prompted me to give up cigarettes for a year. Then I was right back at it, smoking more than ever before.

I'd made a couple of feeble attempts at quitting prior to that. They failed because I didn't have the mindset to quit — I wasn't ready. I tried nicotine gum but it didn't work for me. I hated the chewing. I was teaching school at the time and I didn't want to be chewing gum in front of my students.

When my mother was ill, I started to seriously think about my smoking and the possibility of becoming a non-smoker. Several issues combined to motivate me:

— my mother's illness,
— a severe warning from my doctor about the risks of smoking,
— I knew I wasn't feeling as great as usual and I figured cigarettes were the reason,
— it was becoming socially awkward to be a smoker — I'd go to dinner parties and be forced outside to smoke on the back porch, and
— I felt I was setting a bad example for my high school students.

These issues combined to give me the incentive to become a non-smoker. I wasn't quitting to satisfy anyone but myself. But I knew I couldn't do it alone. I needed help. So I asked my doctor about using the nicotine patch. It helped me immensely, with no adverse effects. Smoking had always served to calm me down. I needed the nicotine that the patch provided. My urge to smoke wasn't nearly as drastic as it would have been without the patch.

I found the withdrawal period difficult for the first six months. My downfall was food. I replaced the soothing effects of cigarettes with food. Before I knew it the weight crept on. If I had to do it over again, I'd stock my fridge with fruits and vegetables and leave the bread and butter alone.

After I'd hit the six-month mark, I felt I'd conquered my habit. I really thought the urge was gone and I was sure I could start smoking socially — one cigarette with coffee after dinner, for example. I was so certain I could keep it under control. I was so wrong. Before I knew it, my habit multiplied. I was smoking more than I'd ever smoked before and I knew

I was no longer well — my COPD had kicked in. I was scared. So I gave the patch another try and, after a tough six-month withdrawal period, I'd quit. Even though I don't think I'll ever lose the urge for a cigarette, I have never touched a cigarette since my second attempt using the nicotine patch.

JEAN'S FIVE TIPS

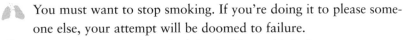

- You must want to stop smoking. If you're doing it to please some-one else, your attempt will be doomed to failure.
- Once you've quit, don't look back. Never think that you can smoke just one cigarette.
- Try medication. I knew I needed help. I couldn't quit on my own. The nicotine patch gave me the boost to stop.
- Be aware that you'll be tempted to replace cigarettes with food. Fill your fridge with healthy things, like fruits and vegetables. Find other activities — I play bridge a couple of times each week — that fill your time and keep your hands busy.
- To avoid temptation, seek out non-smoking environments.

Mychelle's Story

My brother-in-law is a priest. He uses me as an example in his sermons to show how a person can work, struggle, and finally accomplish a goal. He talks about my ten-year battle to stop smoking and the fifteen times I tried to quit. He tells his parishioners about how even someone who is truly addicted to something can finally overcome their addiction — if they're willing to keep working at it.

At least twenty years ago, I decided I would stop smoking. I went to a hypnotist — a doctor in Ottawa — who told me I had so much willpower that it would take ten to twelve visits to get through to me. I had five boys still at home in those days. I couldn't afford the sessions, so I kept smoking.

A few years later, I tried a support group in a local hospital. My hus-band, who was also a smoker, went with me. The instructor specialized in aversion therapy and made us smoke three or four cigarettes in a row, without stopping. I remember the instructor wore a gas mask. At home, she told us to fill a jar with water, put it on the kitchen table, and keep our butts in it. All these things were meant to disgust us. I just thought it was funny. I quit for a week.

At that point, I realized that I wanted to quit but not so much as I wanted to smoke. In the back of my mind, I had a nagging question: "Why should I quit something I enjoy?" In those days, I had no medical problems.

About that time, my father — a man I truly respected — started to ask me why I didn't stop smoking. He couldn't figure out why an intelligent woman, knowing what she did about the health risks, wouldn't give up cigarettes. He didn't understand how completely addicted I was to them.

I kept trying. I tried laser treatments. Didn't work. I bought tapes and listened to them. Didn't work. I went to another hypnotist. Didn't work. For five years, on and off, I chewed nicotine gum. Didn't work. I had two sessions with the nicotine patch. Didn't work. Here's what would happen. I'd stop for a couple of weeks or a month and then I'd decide to "just have one." I couldn't fight the cravings. They were worse than craving food. I had to have a cigarette.

So, here's what made me really stop. My husband died in 1987 and I retired in 1989. I decided it was time to get my financial affairs in order.

MEDICATIONS THAT MIGHT WORK FOR YOU

Smoking is a drug dependency just like heroin or cocaine addiction. We don't usually think of smoking that way because so many of us do it. But across Canada, almost 25 percent of daily smokers take their first cigarette within five minutes of waking, a sure sign of a highly addictive substance.

To give you an idea of how difficult it is to kick the habit, consider these statistics. When asked what would make them stop smoking, 17 percent of Canadian smokers said that nothing (apart from their own death) would make them quit. Although approximately 70 percent of adult smokers want to stop smoking, fewer than 10 percent of attempts are successful. All those relapses are due, in large part, to the iron grip of nicotine addiction. Medication can help loosen that powerful hold. If you're considering attempting to quit, talk to your doctor about using medication.

Two effective stop-smoking medications have been approved by Health Canada: nicotine replacement therapy, and bupropion hydrochloride.

Nicotine Replacement Therapy

Nicotine replacement works very simply. Like cigarettes, the gum and transdermal patch deliver nicotine into the blood. Unlike cigarettes, they don't deliver the harmful toxins that cigarettes contain. Remember, it's not nicotine that causes COPD, it's many of the other four thousand compounds that tobacco and tobacco smoke deliver with each puff. By giving the smoker a steady stream of nicotine, the patch and gum serve to relieve some of the cravings associated with withdrawal from tobacco, making it easier for the smoker to quit for good.

Studies show that nicotine replacement therapies as much as double the chances of successfully stopping smoking when compared with a placebo. Of course, you'll increase those chances even more by combining nicotine replacement therapy with other types of support, like counselling or help from friends. Both the patch and the gum can be used at the same time. And it's also possible to combine nicotine replacement therapy with bupropion. Studies show this combination of medications significantly improves the quit rate over either product on its own.

Many myths surround the use of the patch and gum. Some people will tell you that they're as addictive as cigarettes. That's not the case. Both products deliver nicotine in a way very different from cigarettes. While cigarettes provide the body with a near-instant hit of nicotine, the patch and the gum provide a slow, steady, low-dose stream of nicotine. This means that they have virtually no addictive potential.

There's a common assumption that smoking while using either the patch or gum increases the risk of a heart attack. Not true. The risks of smoking while using nicotine replacement therapy are no greater than the risk posed by smoking alone. Nicotine replacement therapy is safe for smokers and can be used by people who are not yet able to quit smoking entirely. Nicotine replacement therapy may help these people take a "cigarette holiday," or perhaps substantially reduce their smoking as a stepping stone toward successful quitting.

The nicotine patch or gum can be taken as long as necessary to maintain tobacco abstinence. Extended use of these medications over years has been shown to be safe and is much less hazardous than continued cigarette smoking. The nicotine patch and gum are helpful and safe for all smokers who want to quit — even pregnant smokers and heavy smokers under the age of eighteen. Cigarette smoking is infinitely more dangerous.

Nicotine patches and gum are available over the counter in some Canadian provinces. Other forms of nicotine replacement therapy, including a nicotine inhaler and nicotine nasal spray, are available in the United States.

Bupropion

Bupropion hydrochloride, marketed as Zyban, is also prescribed as an antidepressant under the name Wellbutrin. Bupropion's smoking cessation effects were discovered by accident. Because smokers often become depressed when attempting to quit, the drug was prescribed to smokers as an antidepressant. It was discovered that it also alleviated addiction to nicotine. It's still not known precisely how bupropion curbs the desire for cigarettes. We think it acts on the chemicals in the brain in a way similar to nicotine. Like nicotine replacement therapy, it works — doubling quitting rates when compared to a placebo.

It is safe to continue smoking while using bupropion, although smoking while taking the drug appears to reduce the chances of a successful quit.

Certain people should not use bupropion. Those with seizure disorders, or who are suffering from anorexia or bulimia, or who are currently taking another antidepressant should talk to their doctors about these conditions before starting to use bupropion.

I wanted to leave some money for my sons. So I applied for a life insurance policy. That policy cost me an extra $1,000 each year because I smoked. If became a non-smoker for twelve months, I could save $1,000. I gave myself a kick and told myself, "I have lots of willpower. I can do it. I have to do it." But there was more to it. I was starting to notice that my breathing was deteriorating. That scared me. I finally became a non-smoker in 1992 and later that year I was diagnosed with COPD.

Why did I finally succeed? I built on the strength and the expertise I'd acquired in all my other quits. I used what I knew would work for me. I adopted a strategy to handle my cravings. If a craving hit me, I'd get up and do something to take my mind off it — I'd go grocery shopping, drive to the mall, visit a friend. Thirty minutes later, I'd be fine, the craving was gone. I also went back to using nicotine gum. I knew it would give me the extra help I needed. But the most important thing was my attitude. This final time I got rid of the voice in the back of my head that kept asking why I should give up something I loved. I finally faced the cold, hard facts and I became completely committed to quitting.

MYCHELLE'S FIVE TIPS

Treat yourself as an individual. What works for one person won't work for another. Shop around and find the approach to quitting that works for you. For me, I needed the help of nicotine gum.

Fight your cravings. I still have cravings for a cigarette but I don't give in. Instead, I concentrate on something else — I'll work on the computer or throw myself into volunteer work. It's all about changing your patterns and changing your mind.

The decision to quit must come from you. I wanted to quit to please my father but I couldn't. My successful quit came when I decided that I wanted to become a non-smoker — no doubts in my mind.

When you quit, don't criticize those still smoking. I was treated like a criminal when I was smoking. Try to remember how hard it was to quit and show some compassion. Anyway, criticizing someone doesn't work. Support does.

Keep trying. After fifteen quits, I should know.

Smoking Prevention

We spend a lot of effort and thought on helping smokers quit the weed, but preventing young people — or older ones — from beginning in the first place is equally important. Nicotine addiction is probably genetically determined, but at the present time we simply don't understand this well enough to be able to predict who is at risk. It's been estimated that about 60 percent of nicotine addiction is genetically influenced, compared to 40 percent for alcohol addiction and 30 percent for cocaine addiction. This means it's easier to quit alcohol and cocaine than to stop smoking cigarettes.

How much better it would be if we could intensify our energies at smoking prevention for our young people. It's a tough slog, especially when you've got to go up against the slick advertising of the tobacco industry. Kids will continue to experiment with smoking to fit in or protest or be cool (in fact, the teen smoking rate has increased between 1995 and 2000 to a sadly high 30 percent, and 85 percent of those kids started smoking before the age of sixteen). But let's hope they will use their smarts to realize that smoking is ultimately a no-win situation.

And those of you who have COPD can gently use your experience with smoking and its effects to help keep those young people close to you from setting out down that difficult path. Every little bit helps and each individual winner over starting smoking will produce another convert, until the "Marlboro Man" will be nothing but ancient history. (The original Marlboro Man is already history — he died from lung cancer.)

So, keep this fact in your mind: quitting smoking is the single most effective thing that smokers can do to enhance the quality and length of their lives. It's never too late to "butt out"! Yet as Don said at the beginning of this chapter, quitting smoking is probably one of the most difficult hurdles you'll ever face in life. But you don't need to face the challenge alone. Don, Mychelle, and Jean all got help in their battle with the weed — encouragement from family and friends, medication, advice from their doctors. Winning wars — and smoking cessation is nothing if not an all-out battle — is the ultimate test of the capacity of people to work together. Take any help you can get in your fight.

10

"This Stuff Isn't Helping" —
Optimizing Drug Therapy for COPD

If, after you read this chapter, you are contemplating altering the way you take your COPD drugs, or changing the dosages of these drugs, speak to your doctor FIRST!

*B*ecause people with COPD tend to have symptoms (mainly breathlessness, cough, and phlegm) most of the time, both physicians and patients feel it is necessary to prescribe or to take a lot of drugs most of the time. However, it is far better to take the fewest number of drugs possible and to use only those that have a reasonable likelihood of helping to relieve symptoms. You notice we did not say to "cure COPD." You know by now that there is no cure. Once COPD is established, about the only thing that can be done for most people is to treat the symptoms that arise from COPD and to try to prevent and treat complications (pneumonia, COPD flare-ups, etc.). Currently, we simply don't know enough about what's responsible for the development of COPD to devise the drugs that would alter the disease process itself. A huge amount of medical research is currently under way all over the world to try to understand the molecular mechanisms of COPD so that truly disease-modifying drugs can be developed.

Drug Types to Treat the Symptoms

When you think anatomically, you can figure out what you would want lung drugs to do for you. Ideally, you would want a slew of specific medications that would work on the different elements of the respiratory system, drugs that would

— treat the bronchospasm and open up the airways (**bronchodilators**)
— treat inflammation of the airways (**anti-inflammatories**)
— strengthen the breathing muscles (**theophyllines**)
— treat infection (**antibiotics**)
— reduce the amount of cough and phlegm (**mucolytics**)
— treat breathlessness, panic, and depression (**sedatives** and **anti-depressants**)

Several types of each of these classes of drugs are available to treat COPD. The most commonly used bronchodilators are listed in Figure 10.1.

A Note on Drug Names

Drugs come with two names, a **generic** name and a **brand** name. The generic name is the chemical name of the drug, and the brand name is meant to be a sexy, marketable name that will make us all want to run out and buy the drug since it sounds perfect for our needs.

Let's look at the individual classes of drugs you will be using to help manage your COPD.

Bronchodilators

Bronchodilators do what their name implies: they open up, or dilate, the bronchi (bronchial tubes) to help you breathe more easily. They probably accomplish this by improving lung emptying, thus reducing the amount of pulmonary hyperinflation. They may also help by somewhat reducing the severity of coughing. You may recall from chapter 4 that we described a test for bronchodilator reversibility in which the FEV_1 is measured before and after a bronchodilator is administered. If the FEV_1 improves by at least 15 to 20 percent with the bronchodilator, it is assumed that there is some "reversible" bronchoconstriction, and regular bronchodilator therapy is usually recommended.

FIGURE 10.1: COMMON INHALED BRONCHODILATORS
AVAILABLE IN CANADA, 2000–2001

Class of Bronchodilator	Generic Name	Brand Name	Inhalation Devices	Dosages*
Anticholinergics	ipratropium bromide	Atrovent	pMDI (grey with green cap)	2–4 puffs 4–5 times per day and as needed
			Nebulizing solution	1–2 nebules 4–5 times per day and as needed
Short-acting beta$_2$-agonists	fenoterol	Berotec	pMDI (grey with blue cap)	1–2 puffs every 4–6 hours as needed
			Nebulizing solution	1–2 nebules every 4–6 hours as needed
	salbutamol	Ventolin	pMDI (blue with blue cap)	1–2 puffs every 4–6 hours as needed
			DPI (Ventodisk) (two-tone blue)	1–2 inhalations every 4–6 hours as needed
			Nebulizing solution	1–2 nebules every 4–6 hours as needed
	salbutamol (CFC free)	Airomir	pMDI (blue with grey cap)	1–2 puffs every 4–6 hours as needed

Short-acting beta$_2$-agonists	terbutaline	Bricanyl	DPI (Turbuhaler) (white with blue dial)	1–2 inhalations every 4–6 hours as needed
Long-acting beta$_2$-agonists	formoterol**	Foradil	DPI (Aerolizer) (white with blue cap)	1–2 inhalations every 12 hours as needed
	formoterol**	Oxeze	DPI (Turbuhaler) (white with turquoise dial)	1–2 inhalations every 12 hours as needed
	salmeterol	Serevent	pMDI (green with green cap)	1–2 inhalations every 12 hours as needed
			DPI (Diskus) (two-tone green)	1 inhalation every 12 hours as needed
Combination therapy	salbutamol + ipratropium	Combivent	pMDI (white with orange cap)	1–4 puffs every 4–6 hours as needed

pMDI = pressurized metered dose inhaler (puffer); DPI = dry powder inhaler; CFC = chlorofluorocarbon.

* These dosages may be higher than what you are currently taking. They are, however, reflective of published guidelines for COPD management. Always speak to your doctor before making any changes to the way you take your dosages.

** Formoterol is not yet officially licensed for use in COPD in Canada; nevertheless, it is commonly used, and has benefits comparable to those of salmeterol.

It frequently happens, however, that there is minimal or no improvement in FEV_1 after bronchodilator dosing, and yet if the drug is taken regularly there is a noticeable reduction in the degree of breathlessness. How can this be so? The simple explanation is that there is more to breathlessness than FEV_1. It turns out that, in COPD, bronchodilators may be most helpful if they can reduce the amount of hyperinflation of the lungs by improving airflow out of the lungs. But the FEV_1 test is not the most sensitive indicator of lung hyperinflation or of airflow, probably because it is a test that reflects how *forcefully* you can blow air out of the lungs, not how *easily*.

If the bronchodilator helps the airways stay open longer, more lung emptying can occur, leaving the lungs less overstretched. When this happens, the strain on the breathing muscles is reduced and there will be less breathlessness, even if the FEV_1 doesn't seem to change much. The point is that even if you don't pass the reversibility test in the laboratory, you may still benefit from the regular use of bronchodilators with less breathlessness and improved exercise endurance.

NATURAL MEDICINE — IS IT RIGHT FOR YOU?

In this high-tech, complicated world, it's natural to wonder whether your COPD might be treated in a straightforward, natural way. And this thinking forms the basis for many of the natural, alternative, or complementary health care options on the market today.

A wide array of natural medicine options are available, including homeopathy, herbalism, reflexology, naturopathy, acupuncture, and chiropractic, to name a few. Many people believe that these treatments have helped them. But before embarking on any new therapy, it is important to critically analyze claims made for any treatment, whether traditional or alternative. That is, just as it is important for you to learn about your COPD and the traditional ways of treating it, it's vital that you learn the full details of any natural medicine remedy you might be considering.

Often, natural remedies are touted in simple, comforting terms — what could be harmful, for example, about a natural remedy based on common herbs? Well, certain herbs can interact with prescription or non-prescription drugs you may be taking for COPD or other ailments. Other herbs can be potentially poisonous, particularly if taken in large dosages. Take care! Learn about the natural medicine you are thinking of using and ask for proof or evidence that it can deliver on any claims made. The best place to start is by asking your pharmacist or doctor about any possible drug interactions or possible harm that the natural alternative might cause you, and for an opinion on any claims made for the treatment. And remember, you now know there are no miracle cures for COPD. Don't fall prey to false promises.

Bronchodilators are subdivided into two main subtypes depending on how they work in your lungs. The so-called **beta$_2$-agonist broncho-dilators**, such as salbutamol, are so named because they work by combining with receptors in the airways called **beta$_2$ receptors** (receptors are proteins to which the drug must attach before it can do its work). They are **agonists** (from the Greek for contest) because they make things happen. The other main class of bronchodilators is the **anticholinergic** bronchodilators, such as ipratropium, also known as Atrovent. These bronchodilators act by a different mechanism from the beta$_2$-agonist bronchodilators, in that they act to keep the airways open by blocking so-called cholinergic nerves in the airways. Because the cholinergic nerves cause the bronchi to constrict, blocking them with ipratropium results in bronchodilation and easier breathing.

Another class of bronchodilators is the **theophyllines**, such as Theo-Dur (since it has a long duration) and Uniphyl (since only one dose a day is needed). These drugs are actually only weak bronchodilators that nevertheless can be quite helpful in COPD, possibly due to other non-bronchodilating properties they have, such as strengthening the breathing muscles and mild anti-inflammatory properties.

Bronchodilator medications come in short-acting and long-acting forms. The short-acting bronchodilators like salbutamol (Ventolin) and ipratropium (Atrovent) last for only four to six hours, so may need to be taken every four to six hours to maintain their effects. The long-acting bronchodilators on the other hand, such as formoterol (Oxeze, Foradil) and salmeterol (Serevent), last for up to twelve hours, so it is usually recommended that they be taken morning and evening. At the present time there are no long-acting anticholinergic bronchodilators, but it is expected that one such drug, called tiotropium (Spiriva), will be available in 2002 or 2003. This drug is an even more specific anticholinergic agent than Atrovent and seems to have a long duration of action that might help keep COPD airways open all day long.

The onset of action of bronchodilators also varies among drugs. Some bronchodilators (e.g., salbutamol and formoterol) act very quickly once inhaled, reaching near maximum effect within three to five minutes, whereas others (e.g., salmeterol and ipratropium) take up to fifteen to thirty minutes to reach their maximum effect.

How Should You Use Your Bronchodilators?
The sole purpose of these medications is to make you feel better by relieving breathlessness. Since people with COPD are breathless most of the time, they use bronchodilators a lot. You don't have to worry about taking them too frequently. Today's bronchodilators are very safe, and they don't lose their potency if you take them often. You can take as many puffs as you want — within reason.

Contrary to popular belief, if you take more than two puffs four times a day of salbutamol, for example, your heart will not explode and you will not die! We're exaggerating to make a point, but it's common for doctors or pharmacists to tell people with COPD that they should not take any more than eight puffs of these drugs per day; that's the recommended dose. These "rules" come mainly from experience with asthma, and even then they don't have a lot of scientific background to support them.

The reasoning for these recommendations usually goes like this: in asthma, if you can control the airway inflammation by taking inhaled corticosteroid medications (we discuss these drugs below), the airways become much less twitchy and rarely go into bronchospasm. Under these conditions, only one or two puffs of salbutamol, for example, are usually necessary to provide maximum bronchodilation, and since this drug lasts four to six hours, it's not usually necessary to take any more than about eight puffs a day. In fact, if the anti-inflammatory therapy of asthma is working well, bronchodilators should hardly be needed at all.

Furthermore, since these drugs are metabolized, or neutralized, by the body in four to six hours, the maximum-eight-puffs-per-day rule doesn't make sense from the point of view of side effects, either. Beta$_2$-agonist bronchodilator side effects consist mainly of a slight increase in the heart rate and a slight tremor of the hands. If you are not used to taking these medications, even one puff might bring on these side effects, especially if you didn't need to take the medication in the first place. However, if you have been taking these drugs regularly for your COPD, chances are these side effects are no longer a big problem, as they tend to diminish with regular use.

In fact, if you really need these drugs to relieve bronchospasm, it's much more likely that your heart rate will fall rather than rise when you take your puffs. Think about it. When you are battling bronchospasm in your airways, you are working harder to breathe, and so in addition to feeling breathless your heart rate speeds up. When you take your bronchodilator, it works to relieve the bronchospasm, your breathing will become easier, your work of breathing will fall, and consequently your heart rate will fall back to normal too.

These drugs are quite safe and so, if they truly help, you should never be afraid to take whatever number of puffs you need to ease your breathing. The right dose is whatever's enough! For an acute asthma attack in the emergency department, it's not uncommon to be given ten to twenty puffs of salbutamol over a few minutes.

"Not so fast," you say. "I don't have asthma. I've got COPD, so bronchospasm is not a problem for me." You're absolutely correct — COPD is not asthma, so unless you're one of those 10 to 15 percent of COPDers who also have an important asthma component (wheezy bronchitics, or wheezy geezers!), your approach to bronchodilator therapy will have to be different from that of someone with asthma.

Bronchodilator therapy in asthma is recommended on a strictly "as needed" basis, and if asthma management is going well (that is, airway inflammation is under good control), bronchospasm is uncommon and bronchodilators are rarely needed. In fact, recent asthma guidelines state that a sign of good asthma control is to need less than three to four puffs of a bronchodilator per week! When was the last time you felt you could get by with only three or four puffs from a bronchodilator per week? Asthma and COPD really are different. Figure 10.2 outlines the basic differences in the treatment of asthma and COPD.

In asthma, bronchodilators are considered "rescue" medication for bronchospasm. In other words, if therapy to treat the inflammation component of asthma is successful, most asthmatics should expect to be symptom-free most of the time. Unfortunately this is not the case with COPD. Since most of the airway obstruction and damage in COPD is not reversible, people with COPD can expect to be symptomatic most of the time, especially with exertion. COPDers need "rescue" therapy continuously. Since airflow obstruction in typical COPD is there all the time, the benefit derived from bronchodilators is also needed all the time. Thus, for COPD, unlike for asthma, bronchodilators tend to be recommended for regular, round-the-clock use for symptom relief.

How frequently you need to use a bronchodilator depends on how long its effects last. To keep the short-acting bronchodilators like

	FIGURE 10.2: DIFFERENCES IN TREATMENT BETWEEN ASTHMA AND COPD	
Therapy	**Asthma**	**COPD**
Allergen avoidance	Often very helpful	Rarely helpful
Regular inhaled corticosteroids	Essential to good control	Rarely helpful, but often used
Leukotriene antagonists	May be helpful	Not helpful
Beta$_2$-agonist bronchodilators	Rarely needed if inhaled corticosteroids are effective	Regular use may be required for symptom control
Anticholinergic bronchodilators	Rarely helpful or required	Regular use considered by many the first choice for therapy
Theophyllines	Occasionally helpful as add-on therapy in patients on high-dose inhaled corticosteroids	May help reduce breathlessness not controlled with inhaled bronchodilators
Antibiotics for flare-ups	Rarely indicated	Often indicated
Oral corticosteroids for maintenance therapy	Rarely needed	Very rarely needed
Oral corticosteroids for flare-ups	Required for severe flare-ups	Often helpful, but underused

salbutamol (Ventolin), fenoterol (Berotec), and ipratropium (Atrovent) working continuously in your system requires that they be taken four to six times per day. Generally, there is no advantage in setting the clock to wake up for a dose in the middle of the night. If you can sleep through, so much the better! The usually effective dose is two to four puffs each time for any of the short-acting bronchodilators listed in Figure 10.1. This may lead to dosing higher than the so-called daily recommended dose, but the drugs are safe and if you find higher dosing truly helpful, go right ahead.

Anticholinergic bronchodilators seem to be particularly helpful for people with COPD. This is because the destructive process of COPD, especially when emphysema predominates, tends to greatly diminish the

BREATHLESSNESS AHEAD — MAN THE PUMPS!

If there is no major asthma component to your COPD, you need to be a good observer of whether the bronchodilators you have been prescribed are actually doing anything helpful. Remember, bronchodilators attempt to open up the breathing tubes to ease airflow to and from the lungs. However, the increased mucus production in chronic bronchitis and the collapsibility or floppiness of the airways in emphysema also cause airway obstruction, and these conditions are not helped by bronchodilators. Although they do help to open up the airways somewhat, bronchodilators don't have much to work with in typical COPD and so the improvement both in the lung function laboratory and in providing relief from breathlessness tends to be only mild to modest at best.

"Not so!" you say. "My Ventolin helps me a lot!" That may be true, but that response is really more typical of someone with a major component of asthmatic bronchospasm than typical COPD. Consider the following scenario: you've just climbed the stairs from the laundry room and you're all puffed out. So you sit down to rest and at the same time take a few puffs of Ventolin. After fifteen or twenty minutes you start to feel better and move on to your next task. What has happened? Although you may feel it was the Ventolin that eased your breathing, an equally plausible (and often more probable) explanation is that your breathing settled down because you were sitting down and resting, and it was just coincidence that you happened to have taken a few Ventolin puffs. This is particularly likely to be the case if the improvement in breathlessness takes fifteen to twenty minutes to occur after Ventolin dosing, as this drug actually acts within five minutes if there is true bronchospasm to be relieved.

There's another phenomenon working here too. Ventolin, Berotec, and the salbutamol component of Combivent, as mentioned, often have side effects such as a slight tremor of the hands and increased heart rate. Even if these drugs do nothing to help your breathing, these side effects make it seem as if something powerful is happening. So it's important to be a keen observer of whether any of the bronchodilators you take to relieve breathlessness are really doing the job, or whether just resting is providing the main benefit. If rest is more effective at relieving your puffing than sucking on a puffer, you should be able to get by with less drug dosing and thus fewer drug side effects.

Although bronchodilators can be very helpful in COPD, it would be wrong to rely exclusively on them for relief from breathlessness and ignore the benefits of keeping physically fit and of practising an enhanced relaxation strategy to calm down when you're very breathless (see the sidebar "Don't Panic — SOS Breathing for SOB (Shortness of Breath)" in chapter 7).

number of beta$_2$ receptors in the airways, where drugs like salbutamol exert their effect. Furthermore, the daily variation in airway muscle tone or bronchoconstriction in COPD is influenced mainly by the cholinergic nerves in our airways, which act to narrow the airways further, thus worsening airway obstruction. It makes sense, then, that blocking these nerves with anticholinergic drugs like ipratropium (and tiotropium when it becomes available) will help to open up the airways, reducing airway obstruction and thus reducing the work of breathing and the sensation of breathlessness, and increasing exertional endurance for people with COPD.

In fact, many people with COPD, especially when emphysema is predominant, do seem to respond well to ipratropium (Atrovent), particularly when taken in a high dose (e.g., twelve to sixteen or more puffs per day). Why so many puffs? For reasons that were more psychological (read: marketing) than scientific, Atrovent was marketed in North America in a relatively weak (20 µg per puff) formulation. In order to get enough of this medication into your lungs, you must take at least eight puffs per day, and for most people sixteen puffs per day is even better. Taking four puffs of a medication four times a day may seem like a lot, but that's just a throwback to the old eight-puffs-a-day-maximum myth. Atrovent is a very safe medication, with very few side effects, so the biggest problem with this drug is remembering to take it often. When long-acting anticholinergic medications become available, this issue should fade away.

There's another subtle issue with anticholinergic bronchodilators like ipratropium (Atrovent) — there's no "buzz." Beta$_2$-agonist bronchodilators like salbutamol (Ventolin) give you a slight buzz when you take them, a result of the mild side effects of tremor and increased heart rate. When you sense these side effects, you feel that the drug must be really powerful. Since ipratropium doesn't have these side effects, many people think it's not as powerful as salbutamol, even though ipratropium is often more helpful than salbutamol for COPD.

Since salbutamol and ipratropium work by completely different mechanisms, their combined use can result in better relief of breathlessness than when one of the drugs is used alone. That is the rationale for combining salbutamol and ipratropium in the same inhaler: Combivent. Many people with COPD find that taking eight or more puffs of Combivent a day helps reduce breathlessness and improve exercise endurance, without excessive side effects from the salbutamol component. Again, the eight-puffs-per-day-maximum-dosing rule needs to be put in proper perspective. The drugs are very safe, and relief of symptoms is the goal.

Which bronchodilators are best for someone with COPD? It is quite unpredictable whether breathlessness or FEV_1 will improve with bronchodilator therapy, regardless of which drug is used. Some people respond only to beta$_2$-agonist bronchodilators like salbutamol; others respond best to anticholinergic bronchodilators like ipratropium. Some seem to do better when these two bronchodilator types are taken together (e.g., Ventolin plus Atrovent, or Combivent). Still others don't seem to be helped by any type of bronchodilator. The only way to sort this out is to try out the different medications (usually a one-month trial is sufficient) and the combinations to see what works best for you. If you seem to do better without any drugs, so be it. On the other hand, if your quality of life is better with drugs, use them wisely. The endpoint for assessing whether a given bronchodilator is helping you is simply symptom relief: are you less breathless or not? Can you walk farther before having to stop and rest?

If you do respond to bronchodilators, and particularly if you need to take them several times a day, you may be helped by taking one of the long-acting beta$_2$-agonist bronchodilators such as salmeterol (Serevent) or formoterol (Foradil, Oxeze). These are essentially long-acting Ventolin-type drugs that work in your system for up to twelve hours. Instead of having to take your short-acting beta$_2$-agonist bronchodilator four to six times a day, you may only need to take one of these long-acting bronchodilators twice a day. The usual dose is one to two inhalations morning and night. If you usually sleep through the night without breathlessness, you may not even need to take the evening dose.

If you are taking a long-acting bronchodilator, it is still a good idea to keep one of the short-acting bronchodilators on hand to use for quick relief of sudden breathlessness as needed. It does not make sense, however, to continue to take several puffs of a short-acting beta$_2$-agonist bronchodilator a day while at the same time taking one of the long-acting agents. If you notice no difference with a trial of the long-acting bronchodilator, simply stop it, and concentrate on improving your non-drug management of COPD symptoms. At the present time, there is no long-acting anticholinergic bronchodilator available, but when the new drug tiotropium (Spiriva) becomes available, it may provide another helpful treatment for COPD.

There are many pharmaceutical companies making many variations of medications to help people with lung disease and, with few exceptions, all the drugs of the same class do a pretty good job. So there really isn't much to choose between them, and whichever ones your doctor has prescribed will probably be reasonable.

Theophyllines

Theophyllines are comparatively weak bronchodilators available in tablet form. Before the advent of inhaled bronchodilators such as salbutamol and ipratropium, theophyllines were regularly prescribed for people with COPD, but their benefit was minimal and they tended to cause quite a few side effects. So these drugs have fallen into disfavour in recent years and their role in COPD management is limited. Despite this, these drugs have been shown to reduce breathlessness, improve exercise endurance, and enhance the quality of life for some people with COPD.

Theophyllines possess some non-bronchodilator properties that may explain why they seem to help some people, even if no change in lung function can be demonstrated with their use. These non-bronchodilator benefits include an ability to improve the function of the breathing muscles, a stimulating effect on the breathing centre of the brain, an ability to improve the performance of the right ventricle of the heart, and some mild anti-inflammatory properties. Despite these theoretical benefits, most studies of these drugs have shown them to be of questionable clinical significance. Nevertheless, there are clearly some people with COPD who do very much better while taking theophyllines, so it is certainly worth trying these medications if your symptoms remain troublesome despite therapy with short- and long-acting inhaled bronchodilators.

The main problem with theophyllines is the relatively high likelihood of side effects. The concentration of theophyllines can be measured with a blood test, and the maximum benefit from these drugs on improving exercise endurance and breathlessness seems only to occur when the doses are pushed to produce relatively high concentrations of theophylline in the bloodstream. The catch-22, however, is that the higher the blood levels, the greater the possibility of side effects. Theophyllines and caffeine are chemically related, and so the side effects associated with theophylline intolerance are similar to what might happen from drinking too much coffee: nausea, heartburn, diarrhea, tremor, jitters, insomnia, high heart rate, and headache.

Some people are more susceptible to these side effects than others, and it also seems that the older you are, the more likely it is you will experience side effects, even when the blood levels of theophylline are in the normal range. It also stands to reason that if you drink a lot of coffee or tea, the more likely you are to be intolerant of theophyllines. The most severe side effects, usually resulting from inadvertent overdosing, can include seizures, dangerous heart rhythms, and even death.

Theophyllines are best taken in the sustained-release form, which are taken only once or twice a day. To minimize side effects, it may be best to start with a low dose and gradually work up to the recommended dose over one to two weeks. If your breathing gets worse, you should never take extra doses of theophylline in the hope of reducing breathlessness, because the risk of provoking serious side effects is too great. If you are taking theophyllines and they are helping, you should be aware that under certain conditions the theophylline blood levels may increase and produce unwanted side effects. Higher theophylline blood levels may result from the onset of heart failure; the development of liver disease; viral pneumonia; influenza vaccination; or the use of certain medications such as ciprofloxacin (an antibiotic), cimetidine (for heartburn or ulcers), erythromycin (an antibiotic), or allopurinol (for gout).

Newer types of theophyllines are being developed that may improve the symptoms of COPD without the troublesome side effects. Only time will tell how helpful these new drugs will be.

Corticosteroids

Corticosteroids are a class of medication that fights inflammation. They are not to be confused with the anabolic steroids sometimes used by athletes to help build muscle mass. Your own body manufactures corticosteroids in the adrenal glands. These anti-inflammatory drugs are available in oral and inhaled forms; the inhaled forms have fewer side effects than the oral forms.

As we discussed in chapter 2, both COPD and asthma are associated with inflammation of the airways that leads to lung damage. So it makes sense to expect that corticosteroids can help treat both asthma and COPD.

But not all inflammation is the same. In asthma, for example, most of the airway inflammation is due to cells called **eosinophils**. Since corticosteroids work quite well against eosinophilic inflammation, these drugs are the most important therapy for asthma. In COPD, however, most inflammation is due to cells called **neutrophils**, and, unfortunately, corticosteroids do not seem to work very well against neutrophilic inflammation.

So you might expect that corticosteroids are not used very much in COPD, right? Not so! Physicians have a tendency to regard COPD as merely "tough asthma," partly because we do not yet have drugs that specifically treat COPD. The difficulty for the physician is that people with COPD are breathless most of the time. So a lot of asthma drugs, such as inhaled corticosteroids, are prescribed for COPD. At the present time, however, there is very little evidence that inhaled corticosteroids are helpful for the vast majority of people with COPD and could probably be stopped safely in most cases.

Unless there is an asthmatic component to the COPD, the only patients who might benefit from inhaled corticosteroids are those with the most advanced forms of COPD (FEV_1 less than about 30 to 50 percent of predicted), since regularly taking inhaled corticosteroids in large doses (about 1,000 µg per day) may reduce the number of COPD flare-ups for them.

Unlike bronchodilators, inhaled corticosteroids do not act quickly. They are referred to as "preventers." If there is an asthmatic component to your COPD, inhaled corticosteroids should be taken regularly in order to prevent bronchospasm and sudden breathlessness. In either case, these preventer medications must be taken *all the time* in order to be effective. They cannot be taken as needed or only once in a while.

Inhaled corticosteroids may have side effects, so it is very important to determine whether they are right for you. If you seem to be doing better on these drugs, with fewer flare-ups and less sudden bronchospasm, you should take them regularly. If you can't tell the difference, ask your physician about stopping these drugs. If you do take inhaled corticosteroids regularly, the main side effects to be aware of include:

- a sore throat or hoarse voice
- a yeast infection of the mouth (thrush)
- thinning of the skin and easy bruising
- aggravation of cataracts

These rare side effects usually occur only at high doses (more than 1,000 to 2,000 µg per day). Using the lowest effective dose and taking the medication correctly will help to minimize the chance of side effects. If you take inhaled corticosteroids from a pressurized metered-dose inhaler (a "puffer"), all the side effects mentioned can be significantly reduced if you use your puffer with a "spacer" or "holding chamber" (see "Inhaled Drugs Are Best," below). Whether you use a puffer or a "dry powder inhaler" to take inhaled corticosteroids, however, rinsing your mouth with water after dosing will reduce the amount of drug that could be absorbed through your mouth and throat and so minimize the likelihood of side effects.

Oral corticosteroids (such as prednisone and dexamethasone) are rarely needed for maintenance therapy in stable COPD. This is good, since when taken orally for extended periods, corticosteroids can have significant harmful side effects, including high blood pressure, diabetes, weight gain, mental changes, infections, cataracts, thinning of the skin, easy bruising, thinning of the bones (osteoporosis), and necrosis (destructive changes) of the hips. If through trial and error you and your physician have determined that regular use of oral corticosteroids seems to be the only way to make your COPD tolerable, every effort should be made to minimize the chance of side effects by using the lowest dose possible and by trying to get by using an alternate-day dosing schedule. Preventative treatment against osteoporosis (calcium supplements, vitamin D, etc.) is also probably a good idea.

Oral corticosteroids do have a role in the short-term treatment of COPD flare-ups, however, probably because many such flare-ups are driven by an eosinophilic inflammation. This is discussed further in chapter 14.

Inhaled Drugs Are Best

All lung medications, including bronchodilators and corticosteroids, work much faster and have fewer side effects when they are inhaled. This makes sense, since when a lung medication is taken orally, it must first be absorbed into the bloodstream, taking one to two hours before it is circulated to all parts of the body on its way to the lungs. This means that larger doses are required, increasing the likelihood of side effects.

However, when a drug is inhaled, the medication goes directly to the airways to do its work. Much smaller amounts of medication can be used, making side effects less likely. Inhaled medications work faster (minutes versus hours) than when the same medication is swallowed.

That's the good news. The bad news is that not everyone is good at taking medications accurately from an inhaler, because the technique does require a certain amount of hand-eye coordination, especially for the pressurized metered-dose inhaler (pMDI). For this reason a number of different kinds of inhalers and inhaler aids are available.

If you are having trouble with the pMDI, attaching it to a spacer or holding chamber like the Aerochamber can often help. The spacer minimizes the need for coordinating the complex aim-shoot-breathe manoeuvre, making it easier to capture the dose from a pMDI. Spacers also slightly increase the amount of drug getting into the lungs and minimize the amount left over in your mouth and throat. Spacers are particularly helpful when taking inhaled corticosteroids, as they greatly reduce the likelihood of corticosteroid side effects from drug residue left in the mouth and throat.

Another way to simplify taking inhaled medications is to switch to a dry powder inhaler (DPI). With a DPI, there is no jet or spray of gas and medication for you to try to catch. Coordination needs are minimized, since DPI devices are breath-activated. This means that you provide the power to make them work by making a tight seal with your lips on the mouthpiece and then sucking in as forcefully as you can. There are many different types of DPI available. Some come pre-loaded with many doses; others require that you load a dose capsule into the inhaler for each treatment. Some DPIs, like the Turbuhaler (for Oxeze, Pulmicort, and Bricanyl), deliver only pure drug without additives, so there is no sensation that any drug has been inhaled, something that may require some getting used to — it doesn't feel like you're getting anything from the device.

Very rarely, an individual simply cannot use any of the inhalers correctly and must take inhaled medications from a nebulizer using a mask or mouthpiece. This is the way inhaled medications are often given in hospitals, but it is a fallacy to believe that nebulizers are inherently more powerful than simple inhalers. In fact, nebulizers deliver less drug to the lung per unit time (when compared with pMDIs and DPIs), because many of the drug particles they deliver are too large to efficiently penetrate deep within the airways. The only time nebulizers should be prescribed is in those rare instances when use of a pMDI or DPI is physically impossible.

The sidebar "Whistling in the Wind" gives guidelines for correctly using the various inhaler devices.

Other Anti-Inflammatory Drugs

Although non-corticosteroid anti-inflammatory drugs are occasionally helpful in the treatment of asthma, there is currently no good evidence to support their use in the treatment of COPD. These drugs include:

— leukotriene-receptor antagonists (anti-leukotrienes), such as zafirlukast (Accolate) and montelukast (Singulair)
— cromoglycate (e.g., Intal)
— nedocromil (e.g., Fivent)

Drugs Affecting Mucus

The chronic bronchitis component of COPD is associated with continual production of excessive amounts of phlegm. The phlegm tends to be thick and easily infected. It also contributes to the narrowing and obstruction of the breathing tubes and thereby worsens shortness of breath. This excess mucus production is usually the result of cigarette smoke stimulating the growth of mucous glands in the airways, but unfortunately it may not always go away once you quit smoking. As well, because cigarette smoke also damages the airway cilia, the excess phlegm cannot be easily cleared from the lungs, which leads to a chronic cough as the only way to try to keep the mucus levels down ("cough and spit").

Unfortunately, there are no drugs that reliably control or reduce the amount of mucus produced in chronic bronchitis. If the phlegm is particularly thick, drinking extra amounts of water each day may help liquefy the mucus and thus ease its expectoration with coughing.

Antibiotics

Antibiotics are often helpful to treat COPD flare-ups caused by bacterial infection of the airways. However, even though some people with chronic bronchitis regularly spit phlegm that is yellow or brown and looks infected, there is, once again, no good evidence for treating COPD with antibiotics regularly, outside a flare-up. Antibiotics are not helpful for viral infections.

WHISTLING IN THE WIND — INHALER GUIDELINES
Pressurized Metered-Dose Inhalers (pMDIs)

The pMDI is the most widely used delivery system. Similar to other delivery systems, even when used correctly, only about 10 to 20 percent of the per-puff dose reaches the targeted airways. Fortunately, only a small amount of drug needs to be deposited to have an effect.

- Shake the pMDI vigorously three or four times.
- Remove the cap.
- Place the mouthpiece 4 cm (1½ inches, or two fingers' width) in front of your mouth, and open your mouth wide.
- Following a slow, *relaxed* exhalation, start a *slow* inhalation.
- Depress the canister once during the first half of your inhalation.
- Breathe in slowly for about five seconds.
- Hold your breath for as long as possible or up to ten seconds.
- Repeat for the number of puffs prescribed.
- *Note: Rinse your mouth thoroughly after inhaling corticosteroids.*

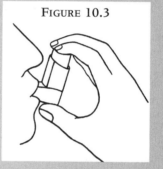

FIGURE 10.3

The so-called open-mouth technique is most often recommended because it is believed that this method delivers more drug to the smaller airways, much as may occur when a spacer is used. However, many people get good results from a pMDI used with a closed-mouth technique, in which the inhaler mouthpiece is inserted in the mouth. (Make sure your tongue does not obstruct the mouthpiece.)

pMDI plus Spacer

Using a spacer with the pMDI can usually assure drug delivery to the airways for most people having difficulty. Several types of spacer are available. Spacers with one-way valves (e.g., Aerochamber) can hold the aerosol discharged from the pMDI in suspension for two to three seconds, thereby easing coordination problems and permitting time to inhale slowly. It is still possible to misuse a pMDI with spacer and miss the dose. Common mistakes include inhaling from the spacer before depressing the pMDI (thus not delivering the drug), and waiting too long after pressing before inhaling (the drug settles inside the spacer). When multiple puffs from a pMDI are prescribed, take each puff separately and wait about thirty seconds between puffs (to recharge the puffer). *Do not* squirt all your puffs into the spacer all at once, or you will not get enough of your medication.

- Shake the pMDI and remove the cap.
- Remove the cap from the spacer, if one is present.
- Insert the pMDI into the spacer.
- Following a relaxed exhalation, insert the spacer mouthpiece between your lips and discharge the pMDI into the spacer once.

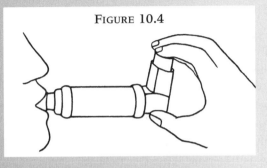

FIGURE 10.4

- Immediately after the canister is fired, breathe in all the way *slowly* from the spacer for about four seconds. A delay of one to two seconds between discharging the drug and beginning to inhale is acceptable. Hold your breath for up to ten seconds, then exhale. For patients with a low tidal volume and inability to hold their breath, taking two or three breaths from the spacer is an acceptable alternative.
- Repeat for the number of puffs prescribed.
- *Note: Rinse your mouth thoroughly after inhaling corticosteroids.*

Dry Powder Inhalers (DPI)
The correct way to use a DPI is device-specific; some come pre-loaded with multiple doses while others require manual loading of doses or dose packs. In contrast to the pMDI technique, a rapid rather than a slow inhalation is recommended for optimum drug delivery.

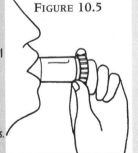

FIGURE 10.5

- Remove any cap from the DPI.
- Load the unit dose according to the device instructions.
- Following a relaxed exhalation, insert the mouthpiece of the DPI in your mouth and form a tight seal with your lips.
- Inhale rapidly from the DPI.
- Hold your breath for as long as possible or up to ten seconds.
- Repeat for the number of puffs prescribed.
- *Note: Rinse your mouth thoroughly after inhaling corticosteroids.*

WHICH INHALER IS WHICH? YOU NEED TO KNOW!
It is important to be able to distinguish among your inhalers. They each have a specific purpose. Inhaled corticosteroids are "preventers," not "relievers" or "rescuers" like bronchodilators, and will not provide quick relief of breathlessness, even if you take several inhalations all at once. Be sure to take the time to go over your different inhalers with your doctor and pharmacist. Most inhalers can be distinguished by their names and colours (see Figure 10.1).

Vaccines

The flu, or influenza, is a viral infection that can cause serious lung problems even for people who don't have COPD. It is a good idea for all people with COPD to be vaccinated against influenza every fall. This vaccination is not 100 percent protective and works only against specific influenza viruses. You will still be susceptible to countless other viruses, which we erroneously refer to as "the flu" when we are unlucky enough to catch one. Nevertheless, getting the flu shot may be one of the most effective ways you can reduce the likelihood of a COPD flare-up this winter. Get one if at all possible.

If you are allergic to eggs, however, you should probably not get the flu shot, as the vaccine is prepared in eggs.

Two new medications may help cut short a bout of true influenza by a few days, if taken within forty-eight hours of the onset of the illness. One of these drugs (zanamivir, sold as Relenza) is inhaled, but is not currently recommended for people with COPD or asthma, since it can occasionally cause bronchospasm. The other drug (oseltamivir, sold as Tamiflu), has not been adequately assessed in COPD patients, so any benefits remain speculative at this time.

There is also a so-called pneumonia vaccination that is recommended once only for people with COPD, among others. The value of this vaccination is not definitively proven for COPD, but it may help and so is a standard recommendation. This vaccine is given only once and will protect against only one common type of bacterial pneumonia, namely that caused by the *Streptococcus pneumoniae* bacterium. You will still be susceptible to pneumonias caused by other bacteria.

Drugs That Modulate Breathlessness

Breathlessness can be debilitating — you know that. Some people with advanced COPD remain disabled by breathlessness despite conventional treatment with bronchodilators, oxygen, and rehabilitation. What can be done to help these folks? In chapter 16, we describe some aggressive treatments such as surgery and home ventilation, but most people don't qualify for, or don't want, such radical therapy.

If breathlessness remains a seriously limiting factor, there is an alternative approach, but it isn't right for everyone, and it must be done with great care. We're talking about sedatives and narcotics — drugs that can reduce the sensation of breathlessness itself. If used carefully and wisely, low doses of sedatives, such as lorazepam, extended-release narcotics such as MS Contin, or even morphine taken as an inhaled medication from a nebulizer, can help "take the edge off" breathlessness and make day-to-day activities more comfortable — without turning you into a "junkie."

If dosages are calculated carefully, this therapy is quite safe. It seems to work best for the "lung fighters" — those people with predominantly emphysema who get very breathless with only minimal activity. The "lazy breathers," who don't have such disabling breathlessness and aren't very active, are unlikely to get much from this form of treatment. Not everyone will benefit from or even want to try this type of therapy; you should discuss it thoroughly with your doctor. A respirologist should also be consulted for an opinion.

Other Drugs

For those rare and unfortunate people who have the inherited form of emphysematous COPD known as alpha$_1$-antitrypsin deficiency (see chapter 2), it is possible to replace antitrypsin with regular injections. This treatment must be given for life and is very expensive. Unfortunately, it is also only minimally helpful for these individuals. Alpha$_1$-antitrypsin therapy is not used for the much more common forms of emphysema.

At the present time there are no other new drug treatments for COPD, but much research is being done in this area as we continue to learn more about the various molecular mechanisms that lead to the development of COPD. The future may hold promise for newer and "smarter" treatments.

Now that you know what is and is not possible from drug therapy for COPD, you might want to consider raising the issue of pulmonary rehabilitation with your physician or even take matters into your own hands by getting off the couch and resolving to become as fit and as active as you can. We assume you've already stopped smoking!

DRUG THERAPY FOR COPD — JUST THE FACTS, PLEASE!

Myth: All people with COPD should take bronchodilators regularly.

Fact: Not all airway obstruction in COPD is due to bronchospasm, so not all people with COPD will respond to bronchodilators. Some do not.

Myth: Taking more than eight puffs of a bronchodilator a day is dangerous.

Fact: Bronchodilators are safe. Many people with COPD can control their breathlessness only by taking sixteen to twenty puffs of bronchodilator per day.

Myth: You should not take your puffers at mealtimes.

Fact: If you take your inhaled medications properly, they should end up in your lungs, not your stomach. Timing them around meals is a non-issue.

Myth: You should take your inhaled medications in the following manner: first, anticholinergics like Atrovent; wait one to two minutes between puffs, then wait ten minutes before taking beta$_2$-agonists like Ventolin; allow one to two minutes between puffs, then wait ten minutes before taking inhaled corticosteroids like Pulmicort; allow one to two minutes between doses.

Fact: If you did this, you'd spend your whole day taking medications. It makes no difference what order you take your drugs in. Nor is there any practical value to waiting so long between doses or types of medications. The best thing you can do is to remember to take all the medications you require, then take them as quickly as possible (holding your breath for ten seconds after inhaling a dose is probably a good idea) and get on with your day!

Myth: Nebulizers are inherently more powerful inhalation devices than pMDIs or DPIs.

Fact: Just the opposite is true: pMDIs and DPIs produce much finer drug particles than nebulizers, so the medications can penetrate deeply into the lungs much more efficiently. In addition, it takes much longer to take a treatment with a nebulizer (ten to fifteen minutes) than it does to get as much drug from a pMDI or DPI (two to four puffs or inhalations). Nebulizers are also much harder to set up, much more expensive, and likely to harbour infectious bacteria if not kept scrupulously clean.

11

"Don't Tell Me I Need Oxygen!" *— Oxygen Therapy*

*O*xygen is a drug and it should be used with the same regard for instructions and precautions as any other medication for COPD. In a way, all of us are on oxygen therapy twenty-four hours a day. We breathe air. That air is a complex mixture of several gases. The most important are nitrogen, which makes up about 78 percent of the air, and oxygen, which accounts for about 21 percent. The 21 percent level is a natural balance that has taken about 4 billion years to achieve. Too much oxygen can cause tissue damage termed **oxygen toxicity**, but that is not a problem with the low concentrations of oxygen in conventional oxygen therapy.

Chronic lung disease can make it difficult for you to get enough oxygen from the natural air into the bloodstream. We call this condition of low blood oxygen **hypoxemia** ("hypo" means low, "ox" is for oxygen, and "emia" is from the Greek for blood). In chapter 1, we discussed how important a safe level of oxygen in the blood is for us: no oxygen = no energy = no life. So with advanced lung disease, it may become necessary to breathe in concentrations of oxygen higher than 21 percent to correct the disease-induced hypoxemia. We call this **supplemental oxygen therapy** or, when oxygen is taken all the time, **home oxygen therapy**.

When COPD has advanced to the point that there is a critically low level of blood oxygen, bad things start to happen. It's like a battery running out of juice. You begin to power down and you feel that you're wearing out: you're fatigued, listless, more breathless. You may not remember as well or think as clearly. All of this comes on gradually over months and years. Many people chalk up this subtle deterioration to the aging process. But if you have COPD or other chronic lung disease, it's a good idea to get your blood oxygen level checked. You may be suffering from hypoxemia, which can often be corrected with more aggressive lung therapy or with home oxygen therapy.

Even though home oxygen therapy can give many people with hypoxemic COPD a new lease on life, the idea of being "on oxygen" is seen as the beginning of the end by many COPD patients. In fact, oxygen can lengthen life, improve quality of life, and sharpen the mental acuity of people with COPD who need it. But you wouldn't know it to hear some people talk.

Peg: "For me, emphysema is gasping old men on oxygen. What a way to live!"

Don: "One of the main reasons I stay off cigarettes is that I don't want to end up on oxygen. Otherwise, I'd say who the hell cares and I'd be back smoking."

Neither Peg nor Don uses oxygen on a regular basis (though Peg was briefly on oxygen after a flare-up).

Now let's hear from three people who have used oxygen on a regular basis for many years.

Lorraine: "I didn't want oxygen. I thought it would confine me. But I proved it didn't. It freed me. I could golf and travel again."

Edgar: "Oxygen is my life support system. Without it, I'd die."

Louise: "Oxygen is no big deal. It's like another piece of clothing that I wear all day, every day. It's become part of my life."

So, we have a medication that's dreaded by those who don't use it regularly and respected by those who do.

Let's explore the world of oxygen therapy with Louise as our guide.

She started using oxygen during a hospital stay in 1997. Since November 26, 1998, she's been using it twenty-four hours a day. During that time, oxygen has progressed from being a necessary evil to just another element of her active life.

"I came home from the hospital in 1997 using oxygen round the clock. My COPD had flared up and the doctors thought I'd be on oxygen only temporarily. Being on oxygen didn't bother me at all. It meant I'd be getting better and then I wouldn't need it anymore," explains Louise. Short-term use of oxygen is a common situation. Oxygen supplementation reduces mortality during acute COPD flare-ups. During a flare-up your body is struggling extra hard to get enough oxygen from the air you breathe. And if you can't get enough oxygen into your blood, the result is hypoxemia.

When lung disease causes your blood oxygen level to fall below a critical value — a PO_2 below about 55 mmHg, or an SO_2% below 88 percent — nasty things start to happen. (For definitions of oxygen level measurements, see information on oximetry and arterial blood gas analysis in chapter 4.) Under these conditions your blood thickens and becomes sluggish because hypoxemia stimulates the body to produce excessive amounts of red blood cells in an attempt to increase the blood's oxygen-carrying capacity. This is called **polycythemia** (too many red blood cells) and it can lead to more viscous blood, sluggish circulation, and a heightened risk of stroke or heart attack. Hypoxemia also means less oxygen for your brain, which can begin to let you down as a result. You may be more forgetful, mentally slow, and even depressed. Correcting this with oxygen therapy can mean more mental energy, less fatigue, and a new outlook on life.

Hypoxemia can also cause problems for both the heart and the lungs. When the lungs are working well, the pressure of the blood circulating through the lungs is relatively low compared to the rest of the body. When the lungs are damaged by COPD and oxygen diffusion is impaired, the blood pressure in the delicate blood vessels of the lung increases. This type of high blood pressure, called **pulmonary hypertension**, is different from high blood pressure as measured in your arm, and it can put a potentially lethal strain on the heart. The right chamber of the heart (the **right ventricle**) pumps blood through the lungs. When you're experiencing pulmonary hypertension, the heart is forced to pump harder to overcome this pressure. If this continues, the right ventricle enlarges and may eventually fail. This condition is called **cor pulmonale** ("cor" from the Latin for heart, "pulmonale" for the pulmonary system or lungs).

Cor pulmonale means enlargement of the right ventricle as a consequence of lung disease. The onset of cor pulmonale is most often gradual. You should suspect it if your ankles begin to swell up regularly and you become progressively more breathless and fatigued. Since cor pulmonale results from the development of pulmonary hypertension, and since pulmonary hypertension is often accelerated by the development of critical hypoxemia, it stands to reason that oxygen therapy may be needed to reverse this process. To determine whether you need supplemental oxygen, your doctor will order tests, including oximetry, or arterial blood gas analysis, to measure the oxygen level in your blood.

LOUISE

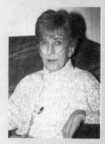

"Attention: Oxygen in Use. No open flame. No smoking." A large sign bearing these words is neatly taped to the front door of Louise's mobile home. And there she is, bustling around, taking coats, and asking if you'd like a cup of tea. Her home is so efficiently organized, you hardly notice she's tethered to her oxygen concentrator by 17 metres of tubing.

She stands for a moment, catching her breath. Then she begins to cough — short, shallow coughs. "I'm not contagious, you know," she says. "It's just my COPD. I tell that to people when I meet them for the first time. If they ask about the oxygen, I'll tell them about that too. I want people to feel comfortable around me, not sorry for me." It's easy to be comfortable with Louise. A lively sixty, she loves to laugh. She's a devoted Elvis fan, an avid reader, and movie buff.

Always bright and capable, she became a registered nurse, married an army man, Deac, and gave birth to a daughter. The family moved every three years, following her husband's military career to army bases across the country. Everywhere they went, Louise landed a job in a hospital.

She loved the life and was always busy and on the move. She enjoyed perfect health. But she had a smoker's cough for years. "Cigarettes were my crutch," she admits. "Hospitals are a stressful place to work. On my breaks, I loved my tea and cigarette. It tasted so good and calmed me down. I knew smoking could cause lung disease, but I thought: 'It's never going to happen to me.' When I'd get bouts of colds and bronchitis, I'd start on an antibiotic. I never gave a thought to quitting smoking."

After Deac retired, the couple moved to Florida in 1986, and Louise worked in an intensive care unit. One weekend in February 1996, she thought she'd come down with a particularly bad case of the flu. She'd been feeling tired, but she'd also been working sixteen-hour shifts. "That weekend I went into hospital and didn't come out for two weeks. I ended up with respiratory failure on a ventilator in the intensive care unit. The doctors told me I had COPD, but I didn't take them seriously until they told

Louise's health did improve during her short-term stint on oxygen, and after a couple of months she was off it altogether. "I was happy to be back to my usual state," she recalls. "I found the oxygen limiting. It really stopped me from leaving the house because I didn't want to drag a portable oxygen cylinder around with me. I had to think about it all the time."

It wasn't long before Louise was thinking about oxygen again, however. "By the summer of '98, I wasn't feeling well. I was tired. I had absolutely no energy and was really short of breath. My colour wasn't good and my ankles had started to swell." These are the classic signs of progressive hypoxemia, pulmonary hypertension, and the onset of cor pulmonale. When Louise talks about her poor colour, she's referring to **cyanosis.** A sign that your blood oxygen levels might be dangerously low is a bluish discoloration of the inside of the lips and tongue. The outside

me I couldn't go back to work. I cried for a week and then I pulled up my socks and thought: 'What am I going to do now?'" She refers to that month in the winter of '96 as "my life-altering month."

The couple returned to Ottawa and Louise began to assemble her support network. She turned first to Deac. "I was suffering from breathlessness and extreme fatigue. I came home from the hospital on supplemental oxygen. I couldn't do anything around the house. Deac did everything." The couple found a family doctor with whom they felt comfortable and who arranged for a respiratory therapist to visit Louise at home and help wean her from the oxygen. She also referred Louise to a respirologist. In 1997, Louise started going to a hospital pulmonary rehabilitation program twice a week. She now goes to a rehabilitation therapy class at the neighbourhood YM/YWCA twice a week.

Louise has kept a detailed diary of her COPD, and it chronicles her many efforts to wean herself off oxygen. "But when I was off the oxygen, I'd spend my days lying down. Everything seemed to be such an effort." Louise has made a truce with home oxygen. She chafes at the limitations it imposes on her life but is grateful for the new freedom it's given her. "It's like an umbilical cord," she says, gesturing to the tubing on the floor and the concentrator sitting in her kitchen. "I feel very comfortable getting around in my own house. Fifty feet of tubing allows me to get everywhere in the house and onto the deck to sit outside. But when I'm using an oxygen travel pack, I'm not as comfortable as I'd like. Still, it's what allows me to get out, travel, and lead a normal life. I have no choice," she states. "If I want to travel, to go to movies, to get out to the Legion, this is what I've got to do."

She's a practical woman who's always done whatever has been necessary to keep her life full and balanced. She just happens to be doing things a bit differently now that COPD is part of her life. "I've chucked the work ethic," Louise laughs. "I used to get up every morning at four-thirty to get to work by seven. Now, I sleep in till nine-thirty every morning, otherwise I can't make it through the day. And I've chucked high heels and bras too. I can't walk in high heels and I can't breathe in a bra. I want to be comfortable. I believe in making things as easy as possible."

of the lips, the nail beds, and the skin may also look blue. (For more details, see chapter 2.)

When the level of oxygen in your blood falls below a critical value, breathlessness may increase. An inadequate supply of oxygen means there won't be enough oxygen reaching the tissues of the body. This lack of oxygen will make every part of you function poorly. Your sleep will be disrupted. You might experience nightmares. As mentioned earlier, swollen ankles is another warning sign that your blood oxygen levels are dangerously low. A low oxygen level not only puts a strain on the chambers of the right side of the heart, it also affects the kidneys, causing your body to retain fluids. The swollen ankles Louise suffered from were the result.

Even though she was feeling ill, Louise resisted going to the doctor. "Looking back, I realize that I was in denial. I thought I couldn't travel if I was using oxygen. I was worried about not getting travel insurance. But I was feeling so unwell we couldn't travel anyway. Everything seemed such an effort that I spent most days lying down." Finally, in November 1998, Louise went to her respirologist, who tested her oxygen levels. She's been on twenty-four-hour oxygen ever since.

By trying a short-term approach to oxygen first, Louise and her doctor chose a commonsense route toward long-term oxygen usage. Typically it's not advisable to decide upon long-term usage during or immediately after a COPD flare-up. Often, as your lungs recover from the flare-up, the need for supplemental oxygen may pass, as it did initially with Louise. If long-term oxygen therapy was prescribed for all people with COPD flare-ups, many people would end up on an expensive therapy they don't really

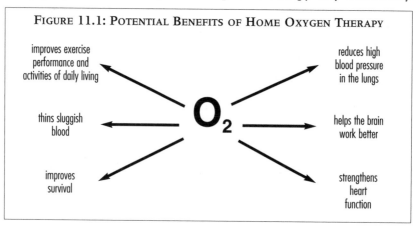

FIGURE 11.1: POTENTIAL BENEFITS OF HOME OXYGEN THERAPY

improves exercise performance and activities of daily living

reduces high blood pressure in the lungs

thins sluggish blood

O_2

helps the brain work better

improves survival

strengthens heart function

need. The decision whether long-term oxygen in the home will help you should wait until your condition has stabilized and you're on maximum medical therapy (except oxygen). Only then should you be tested for long-term oxygen and, if your oxygen levels are still critically low, oxygen should be prescribed.

Although the motherhood statement "oxygen is good" sounds great, it's crucial to realize that oxygen is definitely not a cure-all for breathlessness in COPD. Oxygen will be helpful only if you have critically low values of blood oxygen (hypoxemia). If your blood oxygen is above this critical value (PO_2 greater than 55 to 59 mmHg), breathing oxygen will not do you any good.

When the decision is made to use oxygen on a long-term basis, it must be prescribed in the most effective way. Keep in mind the main purposes of long-term oxygen therapy in the home: the correction of cellular hypoxia and preservation of tissue oxygenation that, in turn, will lead to a reduction of breathlessness and fatigue and the improvement of the quality and duration of life. Once COPD has progressed to the point that blood oxygen levels are critically low, the average life expectancy without oxygen therapy is short — about two to three years. With supplemental oxygen therapy, however, the survival rate in hypoxemic COPD has been shown to improve from about 21 percent at five years to 62 percent at five years.

Oxygen therapy does not cure COPD or reverse lung damage, however, so as time goes on, the impact of lung damage in COPD patients continues. Thus, the ten-year survival rate in hypoxic COPD patients, even when they use home oxygen therapy, is about 26 percent. Nevertheless, most people with hypoxemic COPD using home oxygen therapy will, on average, live six to eight years longer. And, like Louise, their lives can be significantly improved by oxygen usage.

Unfortunately, not all people with hypoxemic COPD respond to oxygen therapy, probably because their pulmonary hypertension is too severe or because they don't breathe the extra oxygen for enough hours each day. We know that the longevity benefits of oxygen therapy will occur only if you use it for a minimum of fifteen to eighteen hours per day, including the hours when you're asleep. That requires commitment. It's important to know that oxygen is not an "as needed" therapy. In other words, if oxygen is prescribed, you must take it for a minimum of fifteen to eighteen hours each day, every day — not just whenever you feel like it. Here's the rule: No oxygen is bad. Oxygen for some of the time is better. Oxygen for most of the time is best.

Oxygen is a drug. If it's determined you would benefit from oxygen therapy, your doctor will usually prescribe oxygen as a **flow rate**, or occasionally as a percentage of oxygen (e.g., 24 percent rather than the 21 percent oxygen in the air we breathe naturally). This flow rate will vary with each individual's needs. Louise's flow rate, for example, is two litres per minute. That means she is receiving oxygen at a rate of two litres of gas each minute. Although Louise's prescription calls for the same flow rate all day long, for some people, flow rates are increased by one or two litres per minute during exercise or sleep.

When oxygen is delivered by nasal cannulae, or "prongs," there is a rough relationship between the oxygen flow rate and the percentage of oxygen you're getting. For each one litre per minute of oxygen flow, the percentage of oxygen breathed goes up by about 3 percent. So, for Louise at two litres per minute, she is getting about 2 x 3 percent = 6 percent extra oxygen for a total of 27 percent oxygen (21 percent + 6 percent).

Your doctor and respiratory therapist will decide on the flow rate appropriate for you. The determination of the prescription for your flow rate is often made with the help of oximetry, and the goal is to raise the blood oxygen saturation ($SO_2\%$) to 90 to 92 percent. (See chapter 4 for more information on measuring blood oxygen.)

When you are starting oxygen therapy for the first time, the flow rate needed to keep the blood oxygen saturation at 90 to 92 percent during

LONG-TERM OXYGEN THERAPY: MYTHS AND FACTS

Myth: Oxygen will help all people with advanced COPD.

Fact: Oxygen will help only those who have critical hypoxemia as a result of COPD. Critical oxygen levels are:

- PO_2 less than 55 mmHg (breathing natural air)
- $SO_2\%$ less than 85 to 88 percent (breathing natural air)
- PO_2 less than 59 mmHg if there is also evidence of cor pulmonale or other signs of hypoxemic damage, such as polycythemia

Myth: Oxygen is a pick-me-up, to be taken as needed.

Fact: Oxygen is useless if taken only as needed. To be effective, oxygen must be taken for at least fifteen to eighteen hours each day.

Myth: Topping up by breathing oxygen for a while before exertion will reduce breathlessness during exertion.

Fact: Not true. Nor will breathing oxygen speed up the time to recover from exertion. Oxygen works only while you are actually breathing it. You can't top up your oxygen reserves. It's not like a savings account.

Myth: Oxygen in the home is dangerous.

Fact: Oxygen is safe. Pure oxygen will not burn or explode. If you use common sense, oxygen is as safe as natural gas heating and cooking. Oxygen will, however, support combustion. What this means is that if you somehow set your oxygen tubing on fire, for example, the oxygen in the tubing will make it (and your nose!) burn faster. This is one of the many reasons for not smoking while breathing oxygen.

Myth: Breathing oxygen will permit you to continue smoking.

Fact: In addition to the fire hazard (noted above), continued smoking leads to a buildup of carbon monoxide (like that produced by your car's exhaust) in your blood and this cancels out the benefits of oxygen therapy, since it reduces the amount of oxygen the blood can carry to the tissues. Smoking while on oxygen is just plain stupid.

Myth: Oxygen is addictive and will lose its effect if taken too much.

Fact: Oxygen is not addictive. You can't become hooked on oxygen. But it's a moot point. If you are chronically hypoxemic, then you need oxygen therapy *for life.* Using oxygen regularly (a minimum of fifteen to eighteen hours each day is essential) will not lessen its effect with time. If you have a COPD flare-up or your COPD worsens, you may need to increase your oxygen flow rates to keep up with your body's needs.

Myth: Breathing oxygen means you will never be breathless again.

Fact: There's more to breathlessness than hypoxemia. Low blood oxygen is only one of the many causes of breathlessness in COPD. Breathing oxygen will help your breathlessness by treating hypoxemia, but it won't have any effect on the other causes of breathlessness, namely airflow obstruction, hyperinflation, and the increased work of breathing. Oxygen will help — sometimes a lot — but it's not the magic bullet for COPD.

Myth: If some oxygen is good, more must be better.

Fact: The correct amount of oxygen is just enough. Increasing the oxygen flow rate beyond what has been determined to keep your SO_2% in the 90 to 92 percent range will usually not help. In fact, too much oxygen can be harmful for some. It's okay to briefly increase the oxygen flow rate for special circumstances, such as extra exertion. If you feel you need extra oxygen in certain circumstances, check with your doctor and your oxygen supply company for advice.

exertion (usually walking) will also be determined. For exercise, often an extra one to two litres per minute above the flow rate necessary while at rest is prescribed. The extra oxygen for exertion may help to reduce breathlessness with exercise and improve endurance. This, in turn, will help you maintain your fitness level, an essential element of good COPD management.

"At first I shed some tears," says Louise of the decision to pursue long-term oxygen therapy. "But I realized that oxygen was going to be part of my life, so I started to learn how to live with it." Her first step was deciding who would supply her oxygen and how she'd have it supplied. Although Louise chose to use the home oxygen provider recommended by her doctor, there were a variety of companies from which to choose listed in the Yellow Pages under "Oxygen Therapy Equipment." Oxygen companies all provide the same products, but it may be worthwhile to shop around. You'll be dealing with the people at the oxygen company regularly — the delivery people and the respiratory therapists, for example — so it makes sense to find a group you like and feel comfortable with and, above all, one that provides good service.

When Louise agreed to accept oxygen full time, a respiratory therapist from the oxygen company contacted her to discuss her needs and assess her physical condition, specifically her oxygen levels at rest and when active. Based on this information, the respiratory therapist recommended the sources of oxygen best suited to

FIGURE 11.2: LIQUID OXYGEN RESERVOIR

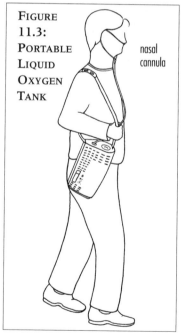

FIGURE 11.3: PORTABLE LIQUID OXYGEN TANK

nasal cannula

Louise. The respiratory therapist told Louise about the three basic sources of oxygen:

- **Liquid:** Liquid oxygen is stored at very cold temperatures in stationary units about half the size of a water heater (like a big Thermos bottle). The stationary unit is refilled by the oxygen company. The frequency of refill depends on the rate of oxygen use. For getting out of the house, small portable units can be filled from the stationary unit. This is a great system for active patients like Louise.

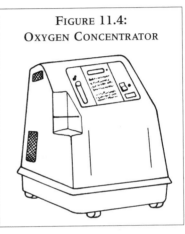

FIGURE 11.4:
OXYGEN CONCENTRATOR

- **Concentrator:** This machine, about the size of a humidifier, runs on electricity and extracts oxygen from room air. It requires some maintenance. For example, the air intake filter must be checked daily and cleaned whenever dirty. This system is ideal for those who are not that active and do not get away from home regularly. Also, users will require a backup system (usually an oxygen cylinder) for when they do go out or in the event of an electrical failure.

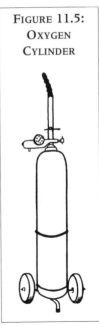

FIGURE 11.5:
OXYGEN
CYLINDER

- **Cylinders:** These metal canisters store gaseous oxygen at high pressure. They can be very heavy and require refilling. Many people use cylinders as backup for concentrators or if they have low oxygen requirements. There are also smaller, portable, lightweight cylinders that can be used outside the home. If these are used regularly, it's best to ask the oxygen company to fit them with a device called an "oxygen conserving device" that acts to prevent oxygen waste, extending the life of the cylinder to several hours.

Louise told her respiratory therapist she wanted to be able to travel, attend movies, go to flea markets, visit her grandson — all the things she'd enjoyed before oxygen. After testing Louise's blood oxygen levels, they decided she'd do best with both a concentrator and a liquid oxygen system. "In the house, I'm tethered by fifty feet of tubing to my concentrator, which sits in the kitchen of our mobile home. I can get everywhere inside the house and even onto the front porch. I have two portable canisters — a four-hour one and a nine-hour one — that I fill from my supply of liquid oxygen and use when I'm away from home."

The therapist visited Louise's home a second time to show her how to operate, maintain, and clean the equipment. "In the beginning, I was a bit overwhelmed by all the equipment the oxygen company dropped off, but the more I worked with it, the easier it became," says Louise. "The machinery is actually very easy to operate. My concentrator, for example — I plug it in, turn it on, clean the filter once a week, and that's it. But you do have to be hygienic about things. The oxygen is administered by **nasal cannula**. Those are the two small plastic tubes that sit at the base of your nose. I clean them every day and get new ones every week or so. It's simple to do, and the respiratory therapist tells you all the details you need to know. If I ever have questions, I call the oxygen company. They're always willing to help."

An example of the kind of advice the oxygen supply company will provide is what to do if your nose gets a little irritated from the nasal cannulae. They may advise switching to a device called a nasal cup that delivers oxygen without the need to insert nasal prongs in the nose. They may also recommend a water-based lubricant to ease nasal irritation, but not an oil-based product such as Vaseline, since there's a risk of the oil droplets being breathed into the lungs, where they could cause damage.

Louise is frank about the benefits and the downsides of oxygen. "Physically, I feel so much better on oxygen. I'm perkier and mentally sharper. My ankles no longer swell. It's what keeps me alive. I would not be able to travel or get out of the house without it. I can do wonderful things with my family. We go to Florida in the winter. I love going to watch the dog races. Of course I never win anything, but we have a lot of fun.

"But it's such a pain to think that something everyone else takes for granted — breathing — becomes such a big deal when you have COPD.

The longer I'm on oxygen, the more I realize that it's the COPD that's the pain in the ass — not the oxygen. In fact, the oxygen allows me to get the exercise that I'd be unable to do without it. I'd be far less fit without it. It's what's keeping me healthy and out of the hospital. Together with my other medications, it's part of keeping myself well."

Louise discovered that it takes time to get used to the emotional impact of using oxygen. "The longer I'm on oxygen, the more comfortable I've become. At first, it used to bother me when I'd be out and people would stare at me. I've realized now that it's human nature to look at something different. Now, I just smile at them. They usually smile back. Actually, oxygen is a great conversation starter. People will come up and talk to you, asking you about it. I still find it hard to be around my relatives, however. They knew me as an extremely capable woman with tons of energy. And I've changed.

"There are definitely downsides to oxygen. Wherever you go, you have to make arrangements. And you always have to think about how long you'll be out because you don't want your oxygen to run out. You can't be as spontaneous. I've learned, however, that the more you go out with oxygen, the easier it becomes and the more relaxed you are with it. And I wouldn't be going out at all if I wasn't on it. Life's not a bowl of cherries — but I'm alive, I've got my family, I travel, I see my friends. I go forward from there — with my oxygen."

12

Off We Go into the Wild Blue Yonder — Travelling with COPD

*T*he meek shall not inherit the earth — especially when they're travelling around the world. Our group proves that travelling with COPD is not only possible, it can be downright pleasurable. But, they all agree, you have to know how to get what you need to accommodate your COPD. You can't be afraid to demand it, if necessary.

JEAN'S TRAVEL TIPS

"Roaming over hill and dale" was Jean's great pleasure as a child. "I inherited my father's love of the countryside — I just can't get enough of it." Unfortunately, Jean learned the hard way that COPD patients can get more than they bargained for from travelling if they don't pace themselves.

In the summer of 1999, Jean spent several weeks on the road. First, she visited her sister in Ireland for three weeks and spent her days touring the country with family members. When she returned to Canada, she headed straight to Hamilton for a family occasion. "I did myself in that summer. I was too active. In Ireland, we didn't have a fixed route. We were staying in bed and breakfasts. Some weren't air-conditioned, some had many stairs. The touring was hard on me. If things started to go wrong — let's say we had trouble finding a place to stay for the night — I'd become anxious and my breathing would worsen. And when you get panicky, you get cross. I'm sure I was a trial for my family," she chuckles. She can laugh now but she found that summer difficult.

"I'll never try a summer like that again," she says. "I've learned my lesson. I have to be careful when I travel and know and respect my limits." Jean will hit the road again this summer, but she knows how to do it right this time.

Be realistic. "I have a bad back plus COPD. I think I've made a realistic appraisal of my health. I know what I can and can't do. Doing things I can't do is no fun," Jean explains. She now knows, for example, that she needs an itinerary in place ahead of time that compensates for her limitations. This will alleviate her anxiety and, in turn, help keep her breathing in check.

Ask for help. "One of the best things I've done on my travels was to ask the airline to provide me with a wheelchair and someone to push it for me," she says. "I thought I'd feel stupid being pushed in a wheelchair but I didn't, and I made all my connections — without being breathless! And all I had to do was contact the airline and tell them I needed help." (You can contact airlines to determine whether you have to change planes en route and, if so, what transportation is available to get you from one plane to the next. Also, you can obtain maps of air terminals from the airport itself, travel agents, or the Internet. Try either www.eAirports.com or www.airwise.com.)

Travel light. "COPD made me reconsider how much I really needed to lug around with me," Jean says. She's learned to pack only the essentials in luggage she can move around without working herself into a breathless state. "I've learned to make do with less."

ARTHUR'S TRAVEL TIPS

According to Arthur, the trick to a successful vacation lies in planning. He's got his vacations down to a science. These days his vacation of choice is a cruise. "I can no longer enjoy the vacations I used to love. Vacations including hiking and swimming are out of the question. Even a golf vacation is impossible for me now. But I've learned to love a cruise. I have a hard time breathing in the cold weather, so my wife, Bev, and I usually take a couple of weeks in January and go cruising in the Caribbean. I plan the arrangements very carefully ahead of time. I examine a map of the ship and choose a cabin in its centre so I don't have to walk the length of the ship. I make certain the cabin is located right beside an elevator so I don't have to worry about stairs. And I always make sure the cabin is air-conditioned and located in a part of the boat that's non-smoking. Then, I sit back and enjoy the cruise."

In the winter of 2000, Arthur and Bev travelled on a Caribbean cruise

JEAN

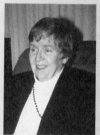

Walking was one of Jean's great pleasures. As a child, she spent her summers exploring the forests surrounding her family's cottage. Her travels as an adult often took her to Ireland to explore and hike. "I could never get enough of the countryside," she says.

Smoking was another of Jean's pleasures. "I'd sneak cigarettes from my mother and father, who both smoked. I really was the worst smoker of all my sisters. I think I may have started the day I was born," she laughs.

Now she's given up smoking, and her walking is limited to getting around the house. Although she's happy to be rid of the cigarettes, she's working hard to regain the ability to walk. In recent years, her COPD has taken a back seat to her back condition. The discs of cartilage that separate the vertebrae in her spine are deteriorating, and it affects her left leg, making walking painful.

Jean, now sixty-four, has tackled her medical issues in a logical, orderly progression, which is not surprising for someone who spent her career as a high school mathematics teacher. She's spent months working with a chiropractor and finally found relief from some of the pain she'd been experiencing. Now that she's becoming more mobile, Jean is interested in dealing with her COPD. She also plans to contact a respiratory therapist to discuss how she can improve her breathing and learn appropriate exercises.

COPD crept up on Jean gradually. When she noticed she was acquiring a smoker's cough back in 1985, she embarked on a campaign to stop smoking. A combination of events motivated her decision with another couple. When the couples were making their arrangements, Arthur was clear about the limitations his COPD imposed on him. He was concerned that, when the ship docked, their friends might stay on board with him rather than hiking around the islands, something that Arthur can no longer do. "I made my situation clear and told them I'd only consider travelling with them if they promised not to hang back with me. They agreed they'd go off and do their own thing. It worked out great for all of us."

Bev is comfortable heading off and touring without Arthur. "During our first couple of cruises, she'd sit with me while our shipmates explored the islands. We decided that was crazy. Now, I'll spend a relaxing afternoon with a book and a beer aboard the ship while she shops and sightsees. I hear about her adventures over dinner."

Before Arthur's most recent airplane trip, his doctor asked him to be tested to determine whether he needed in-flight oxygen. Arthur does not normally use oxygen but he does experience regular bouts of

to quit. She watched her mother die a difficult death from both emphysema and Alzheimer's disease. "Until that point, I thought I could beat the odds with my smoking," she recalls. As more became known about the health risks of smoking, the teacher in her felt compelled to give up her pack-a-day habit. "Being around kids, I didn't want to be a bad influence," she explains. Although still active and working, Jean sensed her health was failing and realized cigarettes were the reason. After two bouts with the nicotine patch, she was able to call it quits.

By that time, however, she was noticing that hiking increasingly made her breathless. "I decided to be tested for COPD, but there was never any doubt in my mind that's what I had." Deep down, Jean knew she had not beaten the odds.

Today, Jean, who never married, lives with her older sister in a townhouse. She retired in 1993 and has spent the years since filling her time with family and friends.

She has unconsciously taught herself how to live with COPD. "I've found different ways of doing the things I want to do," she says. "I take stairs more slowly. I'll sit quietly while my family organizes dinner. I know that if things start to go wrong, I'll become anxious and my breathing will become worse. I'm sure I'm a trial for my family because when you become panicky, you become cross." She's an avid reader, art collector, theatre-goer, and bridge player.

A natural raconteur, Jean loves to talk and laugh. "Talking never hurt me," she chuckles. Getting Jean to talk about her COPD, however, is difficult. "I hate talking about my health," she acknowledges. "And there's a fine line between complaining and informing." Not wanting to cross that line, she seldom speaks of her condition outside a doctor's office. "My friends know me well enough to know when it's a bad day and when to ask me how I'm feeling."

breathlessness. Because the air is thinner in the pressurized cabin of a plane, his respirologist was concerned that Arthur might experience breathing difficulties. Arthur was tested at the hospital using equipment that simulated the environment of a plane's cabin. The testing determined that Arthur would not need supplemental oxygen when flying.

Arthur has his vacation system down pat.

Plan. "If I think ahead and figure out what I'll need and arrange for it, that means I can enjoy my vacation without anxiety. For me, anxiety breeds breathlessness, and I want to avoid that. Time spent planning is a great investment for me." Planning entails requesting brochures and speaking to travel agents to figure out how many stairs you'll face and the best placement for hotel rooms. It means ensuring the places you're staying are smoke-free and air-conditioned. When you're on vacation, it means planning ahead for each day. "We took a resort vacation in Florida one year. I made sure we rented a place that didn't have too many stairs. When I left our room for the pool, I was careful to take everything I needed — my hat, my bathing suit, my sunscreen, my puffers — so I wouldn't have to make return trips to the room. I could just sit and enjoy the sun."

Don't rush — it's a vacation! "Give yourself plenty of time," advises Arthur. "If you're concerned about making tight airline connections, for example, you'll increase your anxiety level, and then it's guaranteed things will become bad. If it's a matter of waiting an hour or two more for a connecting flight — do it. You don't want to spoil your vacation by worrying about running through an airport. You must recognize that you can't do many things as quickly as you'd like when you have COPD. Learn to relax and take things slow."

Talk about your COPD concerns with your travelling partners. If you're travelling with others, be open about your limitations. "I can't do everything my wife can do," explains Arthur. "But we work around my condition to accommodate both our needs. It might mean that we don't do everything together — but we both do what we want and are able to do. And no one feels hard done by."

LOUISE'S TRAVEL TIPS

Florida is Louise's winter destination of choice. "I feel good when I'm there. There's so much I can do: the dog races, walking along the beach, flea markets. I couldn't be outside like that in an Ottawa winter!" Louise is on round-the-clock oxygen therapy. "One of the downsides of oxygen is that it's one more thing to think about before you travel. But the home oxygen companies can make those arrangements very easy for you," she explains. "All you have to do is contact them and tell them where you're going. They'll make the arrangements with an oxygen supplier at your destination."

Like Jean, Louise had made vacation mistakes. Her biggest faux pas was a trip to Phoenix, Arizona. "Because of the city's high altitude, the air was thin. But the worst was the air pollution. I had a terrible time breathing. I was forced to sit inside our air-conditioned condo. Now, before we pick a destination, I ask around about the altitude and the pollution. Florida is great for me — clean air and right at sea level."

Louise is also careful to select a destination with excellent health care facilities. "I'm a nurse, so I'm very aware that I might need hospitalization at any time and I'm also aware that health services vary in quality from place to place. So I check out the services ahead of time." Although this means Louise won't be able to visit certain countries, she'd rather be safe than sorry.

Because of her oxygen needs, Louise is the most careful of our three travellers. She has prepared a vacation checklist that she follows carefully before each trip.

 Arrange for oxygen. Not only does Louise ask her oxygen supplier to arrange for oxygen at her destination, but she also arranges for oxygen while in transit. If she's flying, she'll contact the airline. If she's driving, she'll ask her oxygen supplier to provide the necessary liquid oxygen unit for the trip. Her husband carefully secures the unit into their van with nylon strapping. The oxygen supplier provides all the necessary information about safety, handling, and places to refill the oxygen unit en route.

Get a letter from your doctor. Before Louise plans a trip she visits her doctor just to make certain her health is stable. She asks the doctor to prepare a letter that specifies her condition and her medication plan — information she'll need to communicate if she visits the emergency department of a hospital while away from her hometown.

Arrange medical insurance. Regular travellers' insurance is designed to cover health emergencies, not pre-existing conditions like COPD. Louise makes arrangements to obtain medical insurance tailored to her special health needs and she makes certain that, before she leaves Canada, she's received approval of her coverage from her insurance company. This is an extremely

COPD, TRAVEL, AND OXYGEN — DO YOU NEED OXYGEN DURING YOUR FLIGHT OR AT YOUR DESTINATION?

Ascent in an airplane exposes travellers to what are called **hypobaric** conditions. This means that the air pressure in the plane falls as the altitude increases. At sea level, the pressure of the air surrounding us is about 760 mmHg. Although we are surrounded by this pressure at all times, we aren't aware of it; it's what we are used to. The air pressure around us also influences the pressure of oxygen within our blood (the PO_2). A normal PO_2 in a healthy person living at sea level is about 95 to 100 mmHg. If that healthy person was suddenly transported to the top of Mount Everest, she would be standing, gasping, at an altitude of approximately 8,900 metres above sea level. At that high altitude the air pressure is so low that our healthy person's PO_2 would be dangerously low at about 30 mmHg. This is why Everest climbers breathe supplemental oxygen on the way to the top!

Everest is an extreme but it illustrates the principle of altitude and its effect on oxygenation. You should be aware that if you plan to travel to a place above sea level, it may affect your blood oxygen level significantly, depending on the elevation. For example, Denver, Colorado — the "mile high" city — is perched about 1,600 metres above sea level. In Denver, the PO_2 of a healthy person would be in the range of 84 to 89 mmHg — not too bad and certainly not dangerous. What if you have advanced COPD? Suppose that at sea level your blood oxygen level is 70 mmHg — low, but not low enough to make you feel breathless or cause you problems. If you travelled to Denver, however, your estimated PO_2 would be approximately 55 to 60 mmHg and you might feel quite breathless, especially with exertion, unless you were breathing supplemental oxygen. The effect would be even more dramatic if you travelled to Mexico City, elevation 2,240 metres.

The same principles apply to travelling by air, since the cabins of modern airplanes are not pressurized to sea level but rather to levels in the range of about 1,550 to 2,480 metres.

If you have lung disease, especially COPD, it is prudent to ask your doctor whether you might need to order supplemental oxygen to prevent excessive breathlessness during your flight. As a rule of thumb, if your PO_2 at rest, breathing air at sea level, is equal to or greater than 72 mmHg, it is unlikely that you would require supplemental oxygen during flight. It is possible to estimate what your in-flight PO_2 would be at a reference altitude of 2,480 metres, which is considered the worst-case important step because Louise does not want to end up in hospital in Florida only to discover that she's not insured. Typically, Louise is required to submit a completed medical questionnaire detailing the state of her health before she can obtain insurance.

Pack all the medication you'll need while away. Louise takes along enough medication to last the duration of her trip. Not all medications available in Canada are available in other countries. To ensure her medication gets to the same destination as she does, Louise always packs it in luggage she carries on board the plane. She also packs a medication list from her pharmacist and ensures

scenario when flying in a pressurized cabin. To do this, you need to know your sea-level PO_2 (breathing air or supplemental oxygen) and your lung function (FVC and FEV_1) and do a little arithmetic.

The calculation for estimated PO_2 in-flight is

$$PO_2 \text{ FLIGHT} = [0.238 \times PO_2 \text{ SEA LEVEL}] + [20 \times (FEV_1/FVC)] + 22.3.$$

For example, if your PO_2 SEA LEVEL = 71 mmHg, your FEV_1 = 2.0 L, and your FVC = 3.8 L, your estimated in-flight PO_2 FLIGHT = 50 mmHg. It is recommended that the in-flight PO_2 be kept above 50 to 55 mmHg for your comfort. In this example, you would be advised to have your doctor order supplemental oxygen for your flight. Oxygen must be specially ordered from the airline.

This estimation of in-flight PO_2 is only an approximation, but if it suggests an in-flight PO_2 of less than or equal to 50 to 55 mmHg, breathing one to two litres per minute of supplemental oxygen during flight will likely prevent dangerously low blood oxygen levels and prevent excessive breathlessness during the flight.

It is also possible to simulate in-flight blood oxygen levels during flight using special equipment that mimics an aircraft cabin pressurized to 2,480 metres. This equipment is available only in specialized lung function laboratories. People with COPD who should undergo this altitude simulation test include:

- those with coexisting coronary artery disease
- those who were very symptomatic during previous flights
- those recovering from a COPD flare-up
- those whose blood carbon dioxide level rises when they breathe supplemental oxygen
- those who are nervous fliers

Of course, if you already need supplemental oxygen at home for your COPD, you will need it and a little bit more during flight. The altitude simulation test can also be used to determine how much extra oxygen will be required during flight. In general, oxygen flow rates of one to three litres per minute above what is needed at sea level will suffice during the flight.

that all her medication is properly labelled — just in case. She takes along an extra supply of her medications as well as some "just-in-case" drugs that she doesn't take regularly but keeps on hand in case of a flare-up during her trip. Her extra supply consists of antibiotics and prednisone.

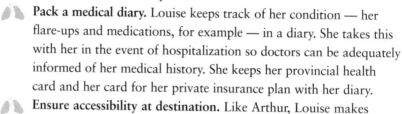 **Pack a medical diary.** Louise keeps track of her condition — her flare-ups and medications, for example — in a diary. She takes this with her in the event of hospitalization so doctors can be adequately informed of her medical history. She keeps her provincial health card and her card for her private insurance plan with her diary.

Ensure accessibility at destination. Like Arthur, Louise makes plenty of phone calls before she leaves to ensure that the places

---

TRAVELLING WITH OXYGEN

The best source of information about travel and your specific oxygen needs is your own oxygen supply company. They can make arrangements for you both en route and at your destination.

At your destination: If you use supplemental oxygen, your local oxygen supply company can arrange for oxygen to be supplied at your destination. To make things easier for you, ask to be provided with equipment similar to what you use at home.

In the air: You and your doctor are responsible for making arrangements for oxygen when you're travelling by air. Be advised that airlines vary on oxygen policies and pricing. Don't assume that because you've done things one way on Air Canada, policies will be the same on Air France.

The majority of airlines will not allow you to use your own equipment; they'll require you to use their equipment. This means you must inform them of your oxygen needs when you're making your travel arrangements. Do this sooner rather than later. Most airlines need at least forty-eight hours' notice of oxygen needs. If you're travelling on Air Canada, for example, your doctor will be faxed a medical clearance document that must be filled out and returned to the airline. Your doctor will provide information about your condition and your prescribed oxygen flow rate. Most airlines charge a fee for oxygen. In 1999, for example, Air Canada charged a flat fee of $100 for all flights. For information from Air Canada's medical desk, telephone (toll-free) 1-800-667-4732.

The airlines will not provide oxygen for ground use in terminals. If you require continuous oxygen therapy, you will have to make arrangements with your oxygen supply company for this portion of your travel.

On the train: Via Rail has size and security restrictions for oxygen cylinders. For example, oxygen cylinders must be secured to the wall of the train car. Check with Via Rail at least three days before your departure to ensure that your equipment meets their requirements.

On the road: Your oxygen supplier can provide you with instructions for securing and storing oxygen equipment in your car. Typically, oxygen units can be secured with a combination of nylon strapping and seatbelts. Do not put oxygen cylinders in the trunk of your car.

she's planning to stay can accommodate both her and her oxygen. She'll ask about stairs, elevators, and proximity of shops and restaurants, for example. "There's no point going if I'm not going to be able to get out of the hotel room," she explains.

With a little pre-planning, travelling can be an enjoyable experience despite COPD. If you have the will, we have the technology to get you there.

NEED SOME HELP?

Our three travellers are great planners. If you don't have the time or skills to plan as they do, there are resources available to help you.

Two **travel health insurance** companies that offer advice on travel insurance are Ingle Life & Health at (toll-free) 1-800-387-4770 and Liberty Health at (toll-free) 1-800-268-3763.

Care Vacations Ltd. is an Alberta-based travel company focused exclusively on arranging vacations — including cruises and land vacations — that accommodate travellers' special medical needs. The company arranges vacations for COPD patients across North America and beyond. Every detail, from oxygen equipment to scooters to wheelchairs to nebulizers, will be organized for you. They'll even train you to use the equipment if you're unfamiliar with it. Care Vacations takes travellers from around the world. For information, telephone (toll-free) 1-877-478-7827, or email stars@carevacations.com.

Oxygen Dependent Travellers' Club of Toronto operates bus trips for those on round-the-clock oxygen and their friends and family. Approximately six times each year, the association travels to nearby casinos, river cruises, or other sites. Oxygen companies supply large oxygen tanks for each trip so the small travelling tanks used by club members can be refilled during the day. A respiratory therapist accompanies the travellers. For information, telephone (416) 438-9656.

Taking Charge of the Air Travel Experience is a guide for persons with disabilities published by the federal government's Canadian Transportation Agency. The guide is designed to help travellers with disabilities plan and prepare their trip by air within Canada. It can be obtained free of charge by telephoning (toll-free) 1-800-883-1813.

The Lung Association offers a wide array of information on travelling with chronic lung disease. This information can be accessed on the Web at www.lung.ca. Also contact your local Lung Association to find out whether there is an oxygen-dependent travellers' club in your area.

Breathin' Easy is a guide for travellers with pulmonary disabilities. It provides more than 2,500 locations to refill oxygen tanks in more than 1,600 cities across the U.S. Plus, the guide can help you plan trips overseas. Contact Breathin' Easy at 225 Daisy Drive, Napa, California 94558 or check out the Breathin' Easy Web site (complete with a chat room) at www.breathineasy.com.

13

Everything You Always Wanted to Know about Sex and COPD — But Were Afraid to Ask

"*I* was a nurse for a long time," begins Louise. "I worked in the intensive care unit of a hospital for years. Many of my patients had serious spinal cord injuries — most of them had been in car accidents. They'd become paraplegics or quadriplegics — instantly. And you know one of the first things they worried about? Sex! But nobody talked to them about it. Most of the doctors and nurses found the topic embarrassing or awkward. The poor patients felt embarrassed too. So I'd try to talk to them. I always started the discussion very gently. 'Has anyone talked to you about sex?' Usually the answer was no. 'Well,' I'd press on, 'sex is going to be different from here on in. But here's the good news — there are ways.'"

So — has anyone talked to you about sex and COPD? Have you asked your doctor or other health care professionals about your sex life? Let's face it. For many — both doctors and patients — it's a delicate subject. It's relatively easy for doctors and patients to talk about the physical symptoms of COPD — breathlessness, wheeze, cough. That's straightforward and easy to measure. But sex is another matter altogether, and so it often gets overlooked.

But not in this book. Louise, who's been using oxygen since 1997, was determined to talk to us about sex. She has no hesitation about discussing her sex life with her husband, Deac. "I fling my oxygen tubing to one side and we go for the gusto," she says with a wicked smile. "In our case, we plan it. We decide ahead of time to have an S&M night," she says. "Oh, it's not what you think! That's a 'sex and macaroni' night. Other nights might be S&S — sex and steak. The key is planning. Sex is not spontaneous for us anymore. But if that's what it's going to take, so be it."

COPD and Intimacy

"I think maintaining a healthy sex life is really important when you have a chronic disease. Maybe even more important than if both partners are healthy," says Louise. "My husband has become my caregiver. He's the one who lugs my oxygen tanks around. He does almost all the cooking and some of the cleaning. It would be pretty easy at this stage of our lives to let everything become drudgery. Neither of us wants that to happen. I want to have a sex life for my own pleasure, but my husband should also be entitled to the pleasure of our relationship. We work at keeping things in perspective, making time for one another. Even if it's just sitting together reading, or enjoying a glass of wine. It's good for the soul and it's good for our marriage.

"COPD doesn't mean the end of your sex life," she continues. "It's the beginning of a new and different life." As Louise mentioned previously, sex is no longer a spontaneous affair for her and Deac. "I make sure that I'm well prepared," she explains. "We like to make a date. That way, I won't plan a day that's overly active. I need to be well rested and relaxed. So that I don't get too breathless, I continue using my oxygen and I also use my inhaler beforehand."

You already know that breath-

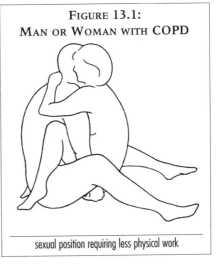

FIGURE 13.1:
MAN OR WOMAN WITH COPD

sexual position requiring less physical work

lessness is a huge deal for partners trying to cope with COPD. You also know that avoiding physical activity because of a fear of breathlessness is one of the worst things you can do. This "couch potato" philosophy only leads to more and more physical deconditioning and, thus, more and more breathlessness. The same philosophy applies to sexual intimacy. One reason sex can disappear from a partnership is fear of breathlessness on the part of either the person with COPD ("I'll die") or the non-COPD partner ("it will kill him or her"). But in reality, studies reveal that average sexual intercourse involves about the same amount of breathlessness as climbing stairs. Of course, it depends on how vigorously you climb stairs and on how energetically you cuddle!

But think about it — it's *natural* to be breathless during sexual intercourse. This is nature's way of telling you that you're doing a great job! It's a fact: the more you become anxious or fearful about the possibility of breathlessness, the worse breathlessness may become. The last thing you need is yet another form of performance anxiety!

Louise has figured out the ideal process for herself and her husband. She ensures she's rested, relaxed, and well prepared. "That way we both look forward to making love," she says. "It's actually very romantic."

Here are some suggestions to help you avoid exacerbating breathlessness and fatigue during lovemaking.

 Rest up. Like Louise, plan to have sex at times when you're rested. If you're better rested in the morning or

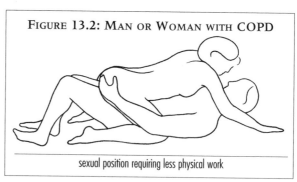

FIGURE 13.2: MAN OR WOMAN WITH COPD

sexual position requiring less physical work

at midday, go for the gusto then. If COPD makes you more fatigued toward the end of the day, don't postpone your intimacy until bedtime. You will enjoy it more if you're awake. If you nap, try a post-nap cuddle.

 Beer, pizza, and sex don't mix. Large meals or excessive consumption of alcohol will contribute to breathlessness during sex. Eat right to play right.

Take your medications. Taking extra inhalations of your bronchodilator before sex may help you to enjoy it more comfortably. This is one of Louise's

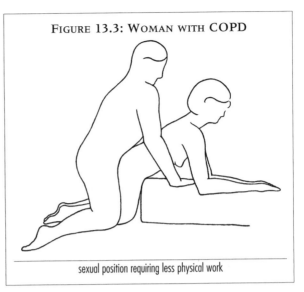

FIGURE 13.3: WOMAN WITH COPD

sexual position requiring less physical work

traditions. Not only does it quell breathlessness, it also helps her keep anxiety at bay. Your COPD medications won't interfere with sexual functioning. On the contrary, they're more likely to reduce breathlessness so that you have the physical capacity to enjoy pleasurable intimacy.

Think about oxygen. Louise continues using her oxygen during lovemaking. If you're already on home oxygen, increasing your oxygen flow rates during sex may reduce breathlessness. If you're not on oxygen but breathlessness prevents sex, consider speaking to your doctor about the possibility of using oxygen during lovemaking. Of course, the best way to figure out whether oxygen will help with your cuddling is to wear an oximeter while you frolic. You can probably arrange to borrow one from an oxygen supply company. If your oxygen saturation level falls much below 85 percent, take this information to your doctor. Oxygen may be helpful, although you will likely have to pay for it yourself, as the provincial governments don't yet recognize falling oxygen levels during sex as an essential indication for oxygen therapy.

Take a rain check if necessary. If you're having a bad day or are unusually breathless before your "date," reschedule your lovemaking. Remember, new or unusual breathlessness may be a sign of an impending COPD flare-up. Get it checked out!

Take a breather. If you've overdone it and are getting too winded, slow down or pause for a bit. Relax, take another couple of puffs of your bronchodilator, then begin again.

Go slow — don't rush! It's not a race. You already know that rushing or walking too fast only makes breathlessness worse. Why would sex be any different? Pace yourself.

French kissing is out. For many people with COPD, prolonged mouth kissing can give them a feeling of suffocation. Nibble an ear instead!

Consider a waterbed. Switching to a waterbed can make lovemaking more comfortable for some couples. By transferring some of the energy of the movement of the water to your bodies, a waterbed can reduce the amount of energy and oxygen you use during sex. The movement of the water moves you without too much effort on your part.

Do things differently — if you need to — and don't feel guilty! Adopt any position that is comfortable and pleasurable for the two of you. The missionary position, with the man lying on top of the woman, supporting himself on his arms and knees, is the most conventional way of making love. But who wants to be conventional? Be creative. Change positions to suit your needs.
If the man suffers from COPD, consider the woman-on-top position, where she can control the pace and rhythm, taking the pressure off her partner's chest.

Maybe you need to completely rethink your definition of sex. Mutual masturbation is another way to avoid breathlessness and still be sexually

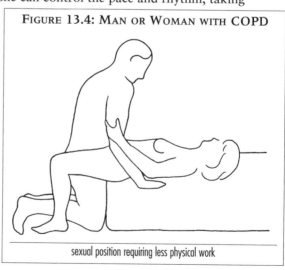

FIGURE 13.4: MAN OR WOMAN WITH COPD

sexual position requiring less physical work

intimate. Even oral sex may do the trick if you're careful about giving yourself enough time to breathe easily.

Although these options may be different from what you're used to, if they allow you to regain a lost intimacy by giving and receiving pleasure, then give them a try. It's important that people who have COPD have pleasurable activities in their lives. They'll feel better for it. And, to quote Louise: it's good for the soul. Throughout this chapter we've diagrammed a few suggestions based on which partner has COPD. Even if you both have significant COPD, lying together on your sides can prevent unwanted pressure on your chests — while permitting pressure on the good bits.

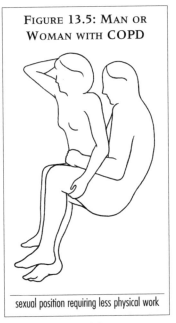

FIGURE 13.5: MAN OR WOMAN WITH COPD

sexual position requiring less physical work

Practice makes perfect. If you're out of sexual shape, don't worry. Have we got an exercise program for you! It's fun and you don't need expensive equipment. But start slowly. Both you and your partner know what to do. Work up to it gradually, and you'll learn new things and relearn forgotten things along the way to healthy sexual intimacy. It's one exercise program you're likely to keep up.

If you listen to Louise describe making a date with Deac for an "S&M evening," it's obvious that the two of

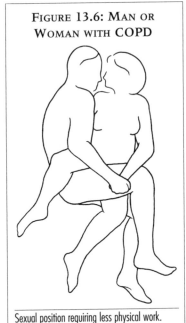

FIGURE 13.6: MAN OR WOMAN WITH COPD

Sexual position requiring less physical work.

them talk openly and honestly about their romantic life. They've learned an important lesson — being open about your needs, fears, likes, and dislikes is probably the most important ingredient in maintaining a healthy sex life. COPD can mean frustrations, disappointments, and fears for both partners. If you don't openly and honestly address those issues first, your sex life will grind to a halt.

What if sex is no longer part of your life with your partner? How do

EDGAR

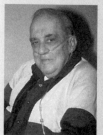

"I'm a dead man walking," states Edgar. And in many ways he's right. At sixty-five, he is in the final stages of COPD. He's now functioning on 35 percent of his lungs' capacity. He has a 60 percent chance of surviving for three years. Since 1998, he's been on round-the-clock oxygen. But that's not all. Edgar's had a host of other health problems, including a heart attack in 1980 and an aortic aneurysm that was discovered in 1995 and repaired in 1999.

Edgar works diligently to cope with his COPD, which is dominated by emphysema. "I spend so much energy breathing, I have little left for anything else. My mind feels that my energy is twenty feet wide, but my body is always reminding me that it's only a half inch deep."

Mentally, it's difficult as well. "I was a policeman. I was into martial arts. I was powerful. I was fit. I'm now confined to my home, hooked up to my oxygen with fifty feet of tubing. I'd love to go for walks with my wife. Yes — I get a little depressed."

But Edgar is not going down without a fight. And he's got a partner — his wife, Marie — who's just as determined as he is. "I've always pushed the envelope," he explains. "If I don't explore all of the options open to me now, I'd feel that I'd let myself down." That attitude has led him to pursue the possibility of lung transplant surgery.

Edgar is a small-town boy. At fifteen, he dropped out of school. Working as an unskilled labourer, he travelled across the country. Eventually, he returned home and became a policeman. Then the big city called and he went to work for the Toronto Transit Commission. He rose through the ranks to become the superintendent of special projects for the TTC's engineering department. He retired in 1990, and he and Marie returned to take up residence in the town where he was raised.

Edgar has two adult children from his first marriage. He always loved sports. His true passions were the martial arts, particularly karate. And, of course, he smoked — forty straight years of a pack or more a day. He stopped smoking in 1990 upon his retirement. "Cigarettes," he says grimly, "were my downfall."

Edgar suffered a heart attack in 1980. "After that, I could still do everything I wanted, but I had to do it more slowly. When I asked the doctor, he said that my slowing down was related to my heart attack. I now realize that it was my lungs acting up. I'd wake up nights and stand by the bedroom window, leaning on the sill, trying to get my air. Once I got it, I'd light up. Like I said, cigarettes were you rekindle that flame? Again, Louise has some interesting ideas. Many of the things she talks about — sitting together and reading, sharing a meal, enjoying a glass of wine, going to the movies together, holding hands, exchanging kind words — are what courting couples do. To restart your relationship, maybe you'll have to go back to square one and begin again. Physical intimacy is a natural product of emotional closeness. It's never too late to reach out.

my downfall."

After he retired, Edgar was plagued by a string of colds. Suspecting allergies, his family doctor sent him to an allergist, who found no allergies but performed a simple spirometry test and immediately diagnosed COPD. By 1994, Edgar was using oxygen on an "as needed" basis.

In 1995, back pains sent Edgar to a chiropractor who, before treating his back, sent him for a routine X-ray. The X-ray revealed much more than Edgar bargained for — an aortic aneurysm, an excessive enlargement of the main blood vessel in the abdomen. For the next five years, Edgar lived under the constant pressure of worrying about when the aneurysm would rupture. He couldn't find a surgeon willing to take on the delicate task of repairing it because his lungs were so bad. He and Marie spent countless hours searching for someone to perform the surgery and finally located a surgeon in Montreal who had perfected a minimally invasive form of the surgery suitable for people with advanced COPD. The surgery was a success.

Now Marie and Edgar have focused their attention on the possibility of a lung transplant. While waiting to find out whether Edgar will be added to the list, they work at keeping him healthy and happy.

Marie is the keeper of Edgar's medical information. Every drug he takes (including date prescribed and dosages) is carefully noted in a sheaf of papers that she carries with her. In addition, she has recorded all of Edgar's hospitalizations, including the details and the names of the doctors her husband has seen in his travels through the medical system. "I never want to be caught unprepared. He's on a complicated regimen right now and I don't want any mistakes to be made," Marie explains.

The couple have organized their home to allow Edgar to exercise daily. They've measured off the hallways of their bungalow so Edgar knows precisely how far he walks each day. Knowing he needs to "put meat on his bones," Marie strives to prepare the most nourishing, high-calorie meals she can for Edgar. "Emphysema is a great way to lose weight," laughs Edgar. "I weighed 210 pounds most of my adult life and now I'm down to 145."

Despite their hardships, life's little luxuries are still a major focus for this pair. Apart from the coldest winter months, they go out every morning for breakfast at a local smoke-free restaurant. In the evening, when Edgar is ready for bed, Marie snuggles in beside him ("I have to make sure I'm not putting a crimp in his oxygen tube," she says.) "We don't talk, we just hold one another. Edgar is no longer capable of kissing. A kiss robs him of his breath. I'm sure this sounds insignificant to healthy people, but it lets us remember our moments of intimacy that were so vitally important to us before this disease entered our lives. These are the things that keep both of us going."

What do you do if you don't have a relationship to restart? For people with COPD, masturbation is a safe form of sexual enjoyment. Many of us were raised to think that masturbation was taboo. In fact, it is an excellent way to provide sexual release and it's much more common than you may think. According to surveys, nearly 50 percent of women in their fifties and 30 percent in their seventies said they masturbate. The numbers are similar for men. We'll say it again — it's important for people with COPD to find ways to feel good and release tension. If masturbation does it for you, great!

What about those couples for whom sexual intimacy is no longer possible? "Edgar is no longer capable of kissing," explains his wife, Marie. "A kiss robs him of his breath. I can't put my arms on his shoulders, around his neck, or near his face because it impairs his ability to breathe." Edgar suffers from severe COPD and is on round-the-clock oxygen. Because of his needs (he now sleeps with the head of his bed raised and finds he wakes with the slightest disturbance), Marie now sleeps in a separate bedroom. Until recently, the couple enjoyed a healthy physical relationship. Now they find it challenging to cuddle for a few moments in Edgar's bed. "But we still make the effort," says Marie. "Although we've lost a lot, we haven't lost everything. We still love one another very much."

This couple's physical contact, albeit limited, is extremely important for both partners. Being together, sharing your love, supporting one another are the truly important elements of intimacy. You're trying to cope with COPD and you'll need help wherever you can find it — a partner, family, a special friend. Intimacy need not be sexual — for some, like Edgar, that simply won't be possible. Marie says it perfectly: "We are intimate on our terms."

Don't hesitate to raise any or all of these issues with your doctor. If you're uncomfortable, consider bringing your partner along to the appointment for emotional support. And remember, COPD or not, it's normal and healthy to have sexual thoughts, feelings, and fantasies at any age.

14

Near Misses — How to Handle COPD Flare-Ups

"Am I going to get better?" These are the words Peg whispered to us as she lay in the intensive care unit of the Ottawa Hospital. During the writing of this book, Peg contracted a lung infection. Her COPD "flared up."

Four weeks after her life-threatening flare-up, we met her at home, where she was curled up on her living-room couch. She was on round-the-clock oxygen. "I don't feel a heck of a lot better," she stated. "I'm still very tired and weak." Two months after her flare-up, however, it's a different story. It's difficult to get in touch with Peg because she's out of the house so much. She's almost back to her old routine of shopping, visiting friends, volunteering on her township's council, and exercising. But she still tires easily and knows it will be at least six months before she's back to her old self. Realizing how lucky she was to have made it through her ordeal, she and her husband, Harold, resolved to make significant changes in their lives to ward off the possibility of a future flare-up and to prepare themselves for the eventuality of another hospitalization. Peg's experiences could happen to anyone suffering from COPD, which makes her story instructive to all.

The Flare-Up

Peg made three mistakes in trying to self-manage her recent COPD flare-up, and the results could have been disastrous.

"I can look back now with perfect vision," begins Peg. "On a Tuesday evening in April, Harold and I went to the casino with a busload of seniors. I had my walker, so I wasn't over-exerting myself. I was coming out of the washroom when I was hit — out of the blue — with the sensation that I couldn't breathe. I hadn't had the flu or a cold, though I had been feeling slightly short of breath in recent days, but not bad. A friend got me a wheelchair. I collected myself and did my pursed-lip breathing. We got back on the bus, and when I got home, I noticed my ankles were swollen and my feet were white — like puffy marshmallows."

"Which she didn't tell me," interjects Harold. "That was her first mistake." Although her feet and ankles were uncomfortable, she ignored them, heading straight for bed.

Two days later, on Thursday, Peg started coughing and spitting yellowy-green phlegm. She discussed this with Harold and both agreed that she needed to start on an antibiotic, realizing that the discoloured phlegm was probably an indication of a lung infection. Peg usually keeps a supply of antibiotics on the ready in her medicine cabinet, but her supply had run out and she hadn't got around to replenishing it. "That was a second problem right there. She didn't get on her antibiotics soon enough," comments Harold. But even then, Peg wasn't feeling too bad and she decided to soldier on. That was her third mistake. She should have seen a doctor immediately.

On Thursday night, she went to a council meeting in her capacity as deputy reeve of the rural Ottawa Valley township she calls home. "My feet were still swollen and I was feeling slightly short of breath. When I returned home, I decided I'd make an appointment and see my family doctor as soon as possible the next day."

Early Friday, Harold drove Peg into town to see their family doctor. She agreed that Peg's COPD was acting up and that she was also suffering from a lung infection. She prescribed an antibiotic (ciprofloxacin) and an oral corticosteroid (prednisone).

Peg was keen to get home because her daughter was arriving from Calgary that evening. After welcoming her daughter, Peg took a bath and climbed into bed. She'd been feeling lousy all evening, but it wasn't until she'd settled in that she realized something was gravely wrong. "I suddenly felt my body go weak. I knew I wouldn't be able to walk if I tried and I was absolutely gasping for breath. It wasn't a shortness of breath that I could handle. It was totally out of my control and I knew I needed help."

Harold called for an ambulance, which, because of their rural location, took forty-five minutes to arrive. Peg credits her daughter with helping her struggle through those long minutes. "She put her arms around me and almost breathed for me," Peg recalls. When the ambulance attendants arrived, they immediately provided Peg with a nebulizer mask and oxygen. That gave her some breathing relief. Finally, she was on her way to the hospital.

Flare-ups of COPD can cause suffering and even death for patients. Some people with COPD seem to be more prone to flare-ups than others, and the frequency of flare-ups is an important determinant of overall quality of life for people with COPD. A COPD exacerbation is a common cause of hospital admission, often following the failure of initial treatment as an outpatient.

It appears that symptoms deteriorate before lung function worsens in a COPD exacerbation. For example, a common prelude to a COPD flare-up is the onset of increased breathlessness, sore throat, cough, and other symptoms of a cold. This goes on for a few days preceding the worsening of lung function. When lung function begins to deteriorate, the COPD exacerbation is in full force, and patients are so symptomatic that they then seek medical help or go to the emergency department.

What is probably happening during the buildup to the COPD exacerbation is the progressive development of airway inflammation. This in turn causes the airways to become more twitchy, leading to increased

---

DEFINITION OF COPD FLARE-UPS

A COPD flare-up or exacerbation is usually defined as a worsening of pre-existing COPD symptoms or the development of new symptoms such as

- new or worsening breathlessness
- new or worsening cough
- increased amount of phlegm
- purulent (thick, unusually coloured) phlegm
- new or worsening wheeze

- symptoms of a cold (nasal congestion, discharge)
- sore throat
- unexplained fatigue or fever

cough and weeping of the bronchi, leading to increased phlegm. All this makes it harder to breathe, and so there is more breathlessness, and, in severe cases, low blood oxygen (hypoxemia) may ensue.

The pivotal role of increased airway inflammation in COPD flare-ups may explain why the early use of a short course of oral corticosteroids, such as prednisone, can significantly shorten the duration of a severe COPD exacerbation and may even reduce the number of flare-ups a person may have over the years. It is not yet common, however, for most doctors to use corticosteroids early on in COPD flare-ups, perhaps because of fear of corticosteroid side effects. Not all flare-ups are bad enough to require corticosteroids. Yet when people with advanced COPD (a low FEV_1) use these drugs for only a few days, the benefits far outweigh the risks.

If the flare-up is serious and prednisone is prescribed, antibiotics should probably also be used, especially if the flare-up is associated with coloured phlegm in someone whose baseline FEV_1 is very low. Remember: you should know your FEV_1 and its percent of predicted value. Having said this, the common association of cough and cold symptoms preceding a flare-up suggests that viral infections of the airways are often contributing factors. You will remember that we said antibiotics are not helpful for viral infections. The problem is that it is very often not easy at all to distinguish between a viral and bacterial flare-up of COPD. Because of this, most doctors favour giving an antibiotic for all but the mildest of COPD flare-ups, especially for elderly people or those whose COPD is advanced.

There are many reasons why a person with COPD could have a flare-up of symptoms. The most common causes are:

- worsening airway inflammation resulting from viral infection, smoking, air pollution, allergies, or bacterial infection,
- flare-up of a coexisting illness (heart failure, for example), or
- unknown reasons. In fact, we don't know what causes one-third of all flare-ups.

Whatever the cause of a COPD flare-up, it can be serious for people with advanced COPD. The risk of dying from a COPD exacerbation that is serious enough to require hospitalization is 10 to 30 percent, and even higher if mechanical ventilation (a breathing machine) is necessary. Being sick enough to require admission to hospital for COPD often indicates the person is quite fragile and has advanced COPD. In one study, for example, the risk of death following hospitalization for COPD exacerbation was

— 20 percent two months after flare-up;
— 33 percent six months after flare-up;
— 42 percent one year after flare-up;
— 49 percent two years after flare-up.

This means that in this study population, almost half of those who had a serious COPD flare-up requiring hospitalization died within two years.

Despite these observations, most people (75 percent) recovering from a COPD flare-up return to their pre-flare-up level of lung function within five weeks. However, for a few (7 percent in one study), lung function had not recovered even after three months. And even though your FEV_1 may return to its pre-flare-up value within a few weeks, it often takes many more weeks for your overall sense of strength and well-being to return to normal — look at Peg.

Hospitalization

"I was so scared when I was in the hospital," Peg recalls. "I never knew what they were going to do to me next. Looking back, it would have helped me enormously to have an understanding of what can happen when you're hospitalized with a flare-up."

Peg's hospitalization was dramatic but certainly not out of the ordinary for someone with COPD. On Friday night, the ambulance headed to a small rural hospital near Peg's home. She was wheeled into the emergency department, and the on-call doctor diagnosed her with **congestive heart failure** ("fluid on the lungs"). He inserted a urinary catheter and gave her intravenous medication called a **diuretic**. By making the patient urinate more, this drug helps remove fluid from the lungs.

Congestive heart failure is the term used to describe what sometimes happens when the left ventricle (the main chamber of the heart) fails because of a weakened heart muscle. If the left ventricle is no longer strong enough to pump the blood around normally, a pressure backup occurs in the pulmonary veins. This results in fluid (mostly water) being squeezed out of these blood vessels into the surrounding lung tissue. It's like filling up a sponge with water. The fluid-filled lungs don't take up oxygen very efficiently, and hypoxemia usually results. It also becomes more difficult to expand and contract the wet lungs with each breath, so the work of breathing increases. The net result is severe breathlessness, fatigue, and low blood oxygen. As a result of the increased pressure, the ankles may swell, as Peg's had. Giving a diuretic (Greek for intensive urination) forces the kidneys to pass more urine (which is mostly water) out of the body, thus getting rid of the excessive fluid in the lungs.

In retrospect, the emergency department doctor was fooled a bit by Peg's breathlessness and swollen ankles. It seemed that Peg's problem was fluid overload from congestive heart failure, and so the doctor started the diuretic medication. But Peg didn't have left-heart failure and so didn't get better with the diuretic. Her real problem was a flare-up of her COPD that caused her to have swollen ankles and troublesome breathlessness. Back in chapter 2, we described how the development of hypoxemia, or low blood oxygen, causes an increase in pulmonary blood pressure that, in turn, puts a strain on the *right* ventricle that can lead to swelling of the ankles. In fact, the left ventricle can be healthy and normal, despite the appearance of puffy ankles. This is what happened to Peg.

The emergency department setting proved daunting for Peg. She was upset when the man in the bed next to her "up and died." Add to this the fact that she had no clue what to expect from the medical staff and was

WHAT COULD PEG HAVE DONE DIFFERENTLY?
Peg has a list of things she would do differently next time:

1. "I'd make sure I had a supply of antibiotics and prednisone on hand and, instead of waiting to see the doctor, I'd start taking them when I first suspected I was on my way to a flare-up. I was too late starting on drugs."
2. "I didn't connect my swollen feet with the condition of my lungs. I now know that swollen ankles can be a sign of a flare-up. Next time I see puffy marshmallow feet, I'm going to run to the doctor." Peg knows she needs to be aware of the physical signs of an impending flare-up.
3. "If I suspected I needed to see a doctor, I'd arrange that immediately. I wouldn't put it off for a day or two. I'd get there ASAP, and if my own doctor wasn't available I'd head straight to the nearest hospital. When I had my flare-up, I told myself: 'I'll be better tomorrow.' I nearly didn't make it to tomorrow because I didn't get to the doctor soon enough."

too exhausted to ask for information. Despite all that, Peg's health seemed to rally. But the next day, she experienced another bout of debilitating, uncontrollable breathlessness. Fortunately, it occurred when her family doctor was present. "I begged her to help me breathe," remembers Peg. At that point, her doctor had only two options to help ease the work of breathing that was quickly exhausting Peg.

One option was to pass a breathing tube down Peg's windpipe (you may have had such a breathing tube if you've ever had a general anaesthetic for surgery) and to hook her up to a breathing machine (a **ventilator**) that would assist her breathing. Doing this is a big deal and requires specialized care, especially for patients with COPD. The other option was to try to temporarily assist Peg's laboured breathing with a ventilator that delivers oxygen under pressure through a tight-fitting breathing mask but without the tube down the windpipe. This is called **non-invasive positive pressure ventilation** (NIPPV) and, when it works, it can rest both the person and the breathing muscles while other therapy treats the cause of the COPD flare-up.

NIPPV is a simpler form of machine breathing (**mechanical ventilation**), but it too requires significant expertise to be administered successfully. The biggest problem with initiating NIPPV is the necessity of a tight-fitting face mask. Although soft, the mask must make a tight seal around the mouth and nose so that no air can leak out. If air leaks, the ventilator can't generate enough pressure to assist the breathing adequately. When NIPPV goes well, the person quickly feels much more relaxed and no longer struggles for breath. He or she is often relieved enough to drift off to much-needed sleep. NIPPV works about 70 percent of the time for COPD. When it doesn't work, one reason is a sense of claustrophobia induced by the tight-fitting mask. This is what happened when NIPPV was tried on Peg.

"I remember screaming to get the mask off me. It was like an extremely uncomfortable football helmet," she recalls. "I couldn't stand the sensation. Then, I don't remember another thing until I woke up in the intensive care unit of the Ottawa Hospital with that machine down my throat," she says.

Harold fills in the missing details. The doctors in their rural hospital didn't feel that NIPPV was working for Peg and felt that she needed to be intubated (have a breathing tube placed via the mouth into the trachea) and mechanically ventilated. Not having the equipment at their hospital, the doctors arranged Peg's transport on Sunday into Ottawa, about an hour's drive from their small hospital.

"I woke up late Monday but I was so heavily sedated I didn't really know what was going on," says Peg. "I did know that I didn't like the ventilator tube and, in my confusion, I pulled it out in the middle of the night. They tried me on the mask ventilation again, but I couldn't cope with it, so I was sedated and re-intubated and went back on the ventilator for another three days. I remember the doctor coming in to tell me they were going to ventilate me. I was dead set against it and told him I'd have no part of it. So he phoned Harold, and when I woke up next I was back on the machine."

Peg wishes she'd had a better concept of how mechanical ventilation works and why it's used before she found herself attached to the ventilator. "About four years ago, I'd had a bad session with my COPD but I hadn't been ventilated. At that time, I told my family: 'Don't ever put me on a machine.' But when I woke up that day on the ventilator, I was so glad I was on it because I still had lots of fight left in me." Harold adds: "I knew that if Peg understood why she was being ventilated, she would

---

PEG'S WORDS OF ADVICE FOR POSSIBLE HOSPITALIZATIONS

1. **Be prepared — with knowledge.** "I spent a lot of time trying to comprehend what they were doing to me," says Peg. She was often too fatigued or "out of it" to ask. Not knowing or understanding the procedures ahead of time made the entire experience more frightening than it would have been if she'd known what was happening.

2. **Be prepared for discomfort.** "Some of the things they'll do to you will be uncomfortable. Try to remember that they're doing these things to get you better and out of there. Keep focused on that — the pain will pass."

3. **Think about whom you want making life-and-death decisions for you before you find yourself in the hospital or an emergency situation. And ensure that that person knows what you want for yourself.** Both Peg and Harold knew that Harold would be her decision maker in the event that she was incapable of making decisions. But if it's not clear who your decision maker will be, decide on someone, let that person know that you've selected him or her, and ensure that you have the proper legal documentation in place. It may be that you need legal advice on that process (see "Tough Choices, Difficult Decisions" later in this chapter). Finally, ensure that your decision maker knows what you want in the way of medical support and is aware of your beliefs and values. You should also speak to your doctor about your decisions on this matter so there will be no misunderstandings if the time comes.

have agreed to it. I knew that when she told us 'no machines,' she meant that she didn't want to be on a permanent life-support system. I knew she wasn't talking about a ventilator that would be used for a short period of time to get her over the hump." Harold felt that Peg was so mentally out of it when she told the doctor she didn't want the ventilator the second time around she couldn't fully appreciate what saying no to the ventilator meant. In fact, it probably would have meant death for her.

Peg was on the ventilator the second time for two more days before her lung disease had improved enough and she had regained enough strength that she no longer needed the assistance of a machine to breathe.

Throughout her stay in the hospital and intensive care unit, Peg's COPD flare-up was treated aggressively by her doctors, nurses, respiratory therapists, and physiotherapists. The presumption was made that her flare-up had been caused by an infection of her bronchial tubes (an acute bronchitis), and so she was given antibiotic medications and corticosteroids, initially intravenously and later by mouth. She was regularly given bronchodilator medications by aerosol through the ventilator, and later by puffers, to try to open up the airways and reduce the effort of breathing and ease breathlessness. Peg was also given regular sedation medication and low doses of morphine intravenously to ease the discomfort and anxiety of her COPD flare-up and of the invasive ventilation therapy necessary to save her life. As soon as she was ready to come off the ventilator, these medications were no longer necessary.

The COPD flare-up had also pushed Peg into a state of hypoxemia. This was one of the reasons for her ankle swelling. To treat the hypoxemia, she was given supplemental oxygen, initially by the ventilator and later by nasal cannulae with a portable oxygen cylinder, which she took home on discharge from hospital. While she was being ventilated in the ICU, Peg was unable to eat, and so her nourishment (necessary to improve her strength) was provided by a thin feeding tube passed via her nose into her stomach. Once she was off the ventilator, the feeding tube was removed and she began to take food by mouth again.

Peg had lots of tubes and "lines" to cope with during her ICU stay. Here's a list:

— **intravenous lines** — for giving medications like antibiotics, corticosteroids, and sedatives

- arterial line — catheter placed in an artery to permit frequent sampling of blood oxygen, carbon dioxide levels, electrolytes, hemoglobin, and blood cell counts and continuous monitoring of blood pressure
- endotracheal tube — breathing tube placed into the trachea via the mouth and connected to the mechanical ventilator
- feeding tube — thin tube placed into the stomach via the nose to provide continuous nourishment
- bladder catheter — thin tube passed via the urethra into the bladder to permit continuous measurement of urine output (important for monitoring fluid balance)
- oximeter — infrared finger clip (like a gentle clothes peg) to continuously monitor blood oxygen levels
- electrocardiogram leads — wires and electrodes pasted on the chest to permit continuous recording of the electrical activity of the heart

Peg was also helped by the constant attention of her nurses, who tended to all her medications and ensured her dignity and comfort. Respiratory therapists maintained and adjusted her ventilator. Physiotherapists helped to improve the strength of her legs and breathing muscles. They were also there when it was time to get Peg out of bed and back on her feet again. Peg was touched by their kindness. "When I was on the ventilator, I couldn't speak to them, but they would come in and talk to me. They all wanted to know why I'm known as Peg when my given name is Bertha. Just hearing their voices took the scare out of the experience. I was very worried about dying. I felt that I was knocking on the door to death. When the doctors would come in and tell me what they were doing and why, it made me feel as if everything would work out for me." Peg was also lucky to have her respirologist as part of the team. Seeing him in the ICU and being able to interact with someone she knew gave her the added confidence that she was in good hands and not just a visiting stranger to the ICU.

Recuperation

"When I first came home from the hospital I thought I'd never get better," states Peg. "They brought me home by ambulance. I needed help to go to the bathroom. I couldn't walk without my walker." But two months after her hospitalization, Peg is getting back to normal and she's worked hard to get there.

A nurse, arranged through Community Care Access Centre, the local community care organization, had been coming in once a week to check on Peg. Those visits have now dropped to once each month. After a month of round-the-clock oxygen, she's tapered down to using oxygen only at night and if she gets herself into a breathing "tizzy." She also keeps an oxygen cylinder in the car in case she needs it when she's out.

Peg knows she's lost a lot of her physical fitness. She kept as active as possible since arriving home from hospital, walking through the house, for example. But she's still out of shape. Realizing she has to work on her endurance, she asked her nurse about the possibility of obtaining help. A physiotherapist, also arranged through Community Care Access, will be visiting Peg's home to start her on a course of exercises tailored to her needs.

Harold rearranged a few things around the house to allow Peg to keep up with her activities. He brought her computer up from the basement, for example, allowing her to keep connected on the Internet and mentally active. Food was a problem at the beginning. Peg had no appetite, but

---

ARTHUR'S ACTION PLAN FOR HEADING OFF A COPD FLARE-UP

This is the action plan that Arthur and his respirologist have put together in the event that his COPD flares up.

1. Try to relieve breathlessness by taking extra doses of bronchodilator (up to two to four puffs every couple of hours, if necessary).
2. *Rest.* Don't overdo it.
3. Drink plenty of fluids and take acetaminophen for aches and pains.
4. If there is worsening or no improvement after one or two days and especially if there is more cough and phlegm, start taking antibiotic and cortisone tablets as directed. Phone the doctor.
5. If at any time during the flare-up you get worse or notice cyanosis of your lips, phone the doctor or go to the emergency department without delay.

This is Arthur's plan and it is specific for him and his COPD. Anyone suffering from COPD should speak to his or her own doctor about developing a personal action plan. For example, not all COPD flare-ups will require an antibiotic or cortisone, but because of Arthur's advanced COPD he and his doctor have decided that he should take both early on during a flare-up. Also implicit in Arthur's action plan is the inclusion of someone who will help out if things get really bad. For Arthur, that someone is Bev, his wife. Your action plan should also include a special someone — a relative or friend — who can help out when you can't cope on your own.

Harold forced her to eat regular meals, knowing she needed to regain her strength. Now, her appetite is back to normal.

She's keeping busy, but on a controlled, realistic basis. "I'm getting outside. But instead of gardening, I'm supervising the work this year and going to garden shops to pick out what Harold will plant." She's been to a wedding but she attended only the reception. Small steps thrill her: she's very proud that she's had a bath on her own and tackled the basement steps. Each day brings a new challenge. She knows that she's got at least four more months of recovery ahead of her. She's determined to progress, and she's not about to make the same mistakes. "Let me tell you — I've become a real nut about checking my ankles," she laughs, vowing to head to the doctor at the first sign of swollen feet.

Tough Choices, Difficult Decisions

At one point during her hospitalization, Peg became incapable of making her own decisions, and her husband, Harold, contacted by her doctors, stepped in. He agreed with the doctors' recommendation that Peg should be intubated and placed on a ventilator as her only chance to survive her COPD flare-up. Thinking back on her hospitalization, Peg wishes she'd been more prepared for the numerous medical choices she and her family made during her hospitalization. It would have made the decision making less stressful during that excruciatingly difficult period of their lives.

You know that COPD is a chronic medical condition. You know that, because COPD eats into your lung reserve, you run the risk of serious ill health, hospitalization, and, possibly, death. What can you do to prepare both yourself and your family?

"You've got to get a grip," states Louise. "That's the first thing. You need to think about the possibilities and then talk over what you want and don't want done to yourself." Louise acknowledges that looking into what may be a medically troubled future is tough, but for everyone's peace of mind, it needs to be done.

You know that sometime you'll probably have to face some serious decisions concerning your treatment in the future. In order to make sound decisions, you need to have good information upon which you base your choices. Medical treatments can seem very complicated, but you need to know the basics to help take the fear and uncertainty out of decision making. To help you out with this, we've made a list of the basic things you should ask about any treatment, whether it be a new inhaler or going on a mechanical ventilator in the ICU. You should have information about

— the nature of the proposed treatments
— the expected benefits and risks
— possible side effects
— alternative courses of action
— the likely consequences of not having the treatments

Where can you get information like this? In many cases, it will be offered to you. If it isn't, begin by speaking to your doctor. Don't be shy about asking specific questions and expecting full and complete answers. If you don't think the doctor's responses are adequate, ask again! You can also gather information from books. Reading this book is a great way to start. Other professionals can help you too. Talk to your respiratory therapist, for example. Since some of these decisions may concern end-of-life issues, they will also involve consideration of your values and religious beliefs, so you may wish to discuss the possibilities with a spiritual adviser or other counsellor. Finally, sit down and discuss what you've learned with your family, or with other people who have had experience with these important COPD decisions.

In the case of COPD, the natural fear is that, at some point, you might end up in a "do or die" situation because of a COPD flare-up or deterioration. Making a decision not to pursue life-prolonging treatment is obviously not an easy one. Usually this decision involves what to do when a life-threatening COPD flare-up occurs. Do you say, "Enough is enough — please keep me comfortable"? Or do you say, "I want to keep going"?

There's no right or wrong answer. The real answer is, It depends. It depends on whether your doctor honestly thinks you can pull through the flare-up and return to your usual life. It depends on whether you like your usual life or are ready to accept that rest and comfort from fatigue and suffering probably means death. It depends on whether you feel you're not done with life yet. You've still got things to do.

The "do" situation usually means a trip to the intensive care unit, where a breathing tube will be inserted into your windpipe (you will be intubated) and you will be hooked up to mechanical breathing machine (a ventilator). The fear is that you may not be able to recover from this flare-up and will end up stuck on the ventilator in order to go on living, which can be an unacceptable prospect for many. In fact, very few people with COPD who suffer a life-threatening flare-up end up dependent on a ventilator. If properly managed, most people can be successfully liberated from the ventilator when the flare-up has subsided and their strength has returned.

Being stuck on a ventilator forever is never a reality unless the ventilator-dependent person with COPD wants to pursue chronic ventilator therapy; some do and it can be arranged, but most do not. If the situation becomes hopeless and there is no realistic chance of ever getting off the ventilator, the person with COPD in collaboration with the doctor and the family can make the decision to stop ventilator support and to arrange a painless, dignified, and comfortable death.

The technology — the ventilator and the ICU — should really not be

WHEN SHOULD I GO TO THE EMERGENCY DEPARTMENT?

Not every bout of breathlessness should send you running to the local hospital. When should you head to the emergency room? You and your doctor should work out an action plan in advance. Your action plan for a COPD flare-up should handle most situations, giving you specific instructions concerning emergencies, and also for dealing with non-emergency worsening of your COPD symptoms. A significant portion of your action plan should contain information and instructions concerning when and when not to head to the emergency department.

If there has been a slow progression (over weeks or days) of your symptoms, there should be enough time for you to consult your family doctor or even your respirologist. The emergency department is for *emergencies* only. It should not be used as a substitute for your family doctor's office.

If you have COPD, the following circumstances may be warning signs of something serious that would justify a trip to the emergency department:

- sudden extreme breathlessness unresponsive to multiple doses of your bronchodilator
- severe breathlessness that has progressed over several hours or even days, despite increased doses of your bronchodilators
- severe chest pain
- chest trauma causing severe breathlessness (with or without chest pain)
- coughing up bright red blood
- a sudden collapse
- a seizure
- the onset of cyanosis of the lips or tongue

much of a factor in the "do or die" decision. As we said earlier, the real decision is whether to draw a line in the sand and not step over it: that is, to make a decision never to resort to mechanical ventilation should the need arise. Although it is not easy, you should give some thought to this question in advance. How you handle this decision will depend on several variables, including your wishes and the opinion of your doctor on the likelihood of a successful outcome of mechanical ventilation — a prediction that is not always easy to make accurately.

Perhaps the single most important issue in this process is your understanding that regardless of your decision you will not suffer. If you opt for mechanical ventilation and it is unsuccessful, or if you decide against ventilation, you will die. But your doctor and nurses, your family, and even you will work together to ensure a peaceful, comfortable, and dignified passing. For some, this will occur in hospital. For others, with planning from your family, doctor, and palliative care team, a restful passing can be assured in your own home.

- a breakdown of your oxygen equipment and progressive breathlessness without any backup oxygen supply
- unavailability of your family doctor, respirologist, or on-call physician, together with progressive chest symptoms

There are plenty of reasons why you *shouldn't* use the emergency department on a regular basis:

- Overcrowding of many emergency departments means long waiting times for non-emergencies.
- Medical attention in the emergency department deals with the immediate problem at hand. Although most emergency department doctors will try to discuss the long-term implications of your disease, their care is no substitute for the ongoing medical treatment you'll get from a family doctor.
- In many situations, emergency department doctors will not have access to your medical records. This could mean that you will be prescribed drugs that duplicate or conflict with your usual medications. (You should always go to the emergency department with all of the drugs you are currently taking.)
- Communication between the emergency department and your family doctor may not be perfect. This means the onus is on you to ask for a copy of your emergency department record to take home. After a visit to the emergency department, report back to your family doctor and provide a record of your treatment.

Everyone gets frightened when they can't breathe. That's why it makes good sense to calm your fears by understanding what a true COPD emergency is and having a plan in place to deal with an emergency, if one ever arises in your life.

End-of-life issues are complex and there is another important issue to consider. What if you become incapacitated and cannot make decisions on your own behalf, even if only temporarily? Peg was temporarily incapacitated during her flare-up. In a situation of mental incapacity, no one, not even your spouse, has the automatic legal right to make decisions on your behalf. To prevent any confusion down the road, it makes very good sense to do some upfront planning. Creating your own power of attorney for personal care is one of the easiest ways to do this. That's what Louise has done. Plus, she's taken the time to sit down with her husband and only daughter to talk about her future and the decisions they may have to make about her life.

Powers of Attorney for Personal Care and Living Wills

A power of attorney for personal care is a legal document authorizing one or more people to make personal care decisions for you if you ever become mentally incapable of making those decisions yourself. In the power of attorney, you can give instructions about all aspects of your life, including where you want to live, what you want to wear, and what kind of medical treatment you want. Although it can be a very simple document, there are legal restrictions on its format. To ensure it's legally binding, get it reviewed by a lawyer.

There are a number of issues to consider when preparing a power of attorney for personal care:

Who will you choose? Who will you choose to make all those decisions on your behalf? You want someone you can trust and who knows you well. You'll obviously want to talk with the person you've chosen. Maybe he or she doesn't want the responsibility. Discuss your instructions and how you want them carried out.

What will your instructions be? Your instructions can be extraordinarily detailed or non-existent. You don't have to give any instructions for your care in your power of attorney if you choose not to. In this case, your attorney — the person you choose to make your decisions — can make decisions as best as he or she can in any given situation. If you opt for this approach, you're going to want to make sure you've talked in advance with your chosen person about your wishes and values. On the other hand, you can make your instructions as detailed as you'd like. For example, you can attach a **living will**, also known as **advance medical directives**, to your power of attorney. In a living will, you specify the types of medical treatment you choose or refuse. For instance, you might specify that you don't want to be kept alive on a life support system.

We offer a few words of warning here. In Peg's experience, she needed to be hooked up to many machines, but only for a couple of days until her flare-up had passed. You might say you don't want to be hooked up to a life support system. But what if you needed it only for a couple of days? Explain your instructions: "I don't want to be hooked up to a machine if I'll be dependent on it for the rest of my natural life." Similarly, be clear and specific. Be aware of the different degrees of your illness. If you have a serious flare-up that could leave you permanently mentally incapacitated, you might give instructions about your long-term care different from what you would if you have a flare-up from which you'll recover fully within a few weeks (as Peg had).

In her power of attorney for personal care, Louise has taken a balanced approach between no instructions and reams of details. Understanding that medications and treatments change and improve, Louise doesn't want to get caught by overly specific instructions that could result in her premature death. Understanding that written words can never replace a frank discussion, and that she can never possibly anticipate all the decisions her family may need to make on her behalf, she has opted for simple instructions combined with an ongoing series of conversations with her husband and daughter about her values and wishes.

15

A Brief Tour of Other Lung Diseases

Why are we including information on *other* lung diseases in a book about COPD? Well, as Raymond says, "Education is your friend," and he's right. Although most lung diseases lead to the common symptoms of breathlessness, cough, and excess phlegm, each has different causes and treatments. It's helpful to know about other lung diseases, especially if you're wondering whether your COPD might be complicated by the presence of another lung disease. Also, the terminology of lung disease can be confusing and is not always used accurately, even by doctors and other health professionals.

Doctors can sometimes be short on specifics when talking to their patients. If your doctor's diagnosis is vague ("You have an obstructive lung disease"), don't hesitate to ask for clarification. Ask whether you have any elements of other lung diseases — asthma, for example. Never hesitate to insist on a specific diagnosis of your disease.

Common areas of confusion for doctors and patients are "asthma versus COPD" and "chronic bronchitis versus emphysema." In fact, all of these conditions can overlap within the same individual. A basic understanding of the similarities and differences can often help to clear the air. So, let's review the basics. As you know from reading chapter 2, lung diseases usually fall into one of two categories — obstructive and restrictive.

Obstructive Lung Diseases Other Than COPD

Asthma

Church can be a dangerous place for Arthur. "If I'm sitting beside someone drenched in perfume or aftershave, I've got to move. Actually, any strong odour — the scent of flowers, for example — will tighten my chest up. Before you know it, I'm working to catch my breath." Arthur's reaction to scents reveals that, on top of his COPD, he's also suffering from asthma with bronchial hyper-responsiveness. But what is asthma, anyway?

Think about having a cold. Your nose is stuffed up. You're having trouble breathing because your nasal passages are swollen and sensitive. Your pockets are full of balled-up tissues. Your doctor will tell you the inside of your nose is inflamed. That's what happens in asthma — it's like having a head cold in your lungs. Throw in some chest tightness and wheezy breathlessness for good measure and keep it going for twenty-four hours a day. Add an on/off switch over which you seem to have no control. Turned on, that switch triggers your air passages to twitch and tighten, causing you to cough and wheeze. That's asthma.

Predisposition for asthma is probably genetically determined. The end result is injured airways. The injury can begin in numerous ways. If you are unlucky enough to be genetically predisposed to asthma, your airways are prone to develop a form of persisting inflammation. **Inflammation** is that puffy redness you see surrounding a cut. It's often warm to the touch and it weeps. Touch it and it hurts. When bronchial tubes are disturbed by inflammation, they go into spasm — **bronchospasm**. The combination of bronchospasm plus inflamed, weepy, narrowed airways makes asthma one of the big two obstructive lung diseases. (The other, of course, is COPD.)

Because asthma is a disease that narrows the air passages, it is difficult for asthmatics to get air out of the lungs. But that's not how it feels to most asthmatics (or to those with COPD, for that matter). Surprisingly, most complain of the uncomfortable feeling of not being able to get

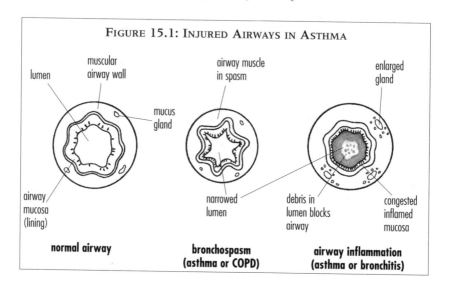

FIGURE 15.1: INJURED AIRWAYS IN ASTHMA

muscular airway wall · lumen · mucus gland · airway muscle in spasm · enlarged gland · airway mucosa (lining) · narrowed lumen · debris in lumen blocks airway · congested inflamed mucosa

normal airway · **bronchospasm (asthma or COPD)** · **airway inflammation (asthma or bronchitis)**

enough air *into* their lungs. The reason is hyperinflation, as we discussed in chapter 2. The air in the asthmatic's lungs becomes trapped behind the narrowed air passages so that there's no more room to inhale fresh air. The result is horrible breathlessness.

When bronchospasm occurs, the asthmatic also has to cope with the sensation of having a very tight chest. It feels like the elasticity is gone from your chest. When you take a breath in, you feel like you're using only the top little bit of your lungs. It's a stressful feeling and becomes ever more stressful because, in your head, you're trying to concentrate on breathing and relaxing. But when you're fighting for every breath, that's easier said than done. People with advanced COPD feel the same way, but the causes are often different, and in COPD, because the light switch is always on, the fighting never stops.

Telling the Difference between COPD and Asthma

Although COPD and asthma often produce similar symptoms of cough, breathlessness, and wheeze, they are quite different conditions and respond differently to various pulmonary medications. It's important to distinguish between asthma and COPD, because both treatment and prognosis are different for each disorder. Asthma and COPD are both examples of obstructive lung diseases, and both are associated with airway inflammation, but the type of inflammation is different in each.

In asthma, the airway inflammation is driven by cells called **eosinophils**. In COPD, cells called **neutrophils** and **macrophages** seem to be the main culprits. This difference influences treatment. The eosinophilic inflammation of asthma responds well to treatment with corticosteroid medications, whereas the neutrophilic inflammation of COPD is less responsive to these drugs.

About 10 to 15 percent of smokers or former smokers with COPD may also have elements of asthma. This group is often referred to as having **wheezy bronchitis**. Although not absolute, the features that may help differentiate COPD from asthma are listed in Figure 15.2.

Asthma is characterized by a more intermittent behaviour than COPD. Asthma symptoms and bronchospasm are worse when the eosinophilic inflammation is not well controlled. They can usually be improved by adjusting drug therapy. When asthma is under good control, symptoms are minimal or even absent. This on-and-off behaviour of asthma is often termed **airway hyper-responsiveness**. This means the airways of asthmatics are irritable or "twitchy." When exposed to an asthma trigger (a pet cat or a strong odour, for example), the asthmatic's airways can get more inflamed and go into bronchospasm, leading to chest tightness and breathlessness. When the exposure is over and the inflammation is brought under control, the airways calm down and are not so irritable.

Asthmatics need to be aware of those things that can trigger an asthma attack or flare-up. Different people have different triggers. Some asthmatics seem to have trouble with asthma only when they have a viral infection of the airways (a cold). Others have allergic triggering factors, such as exposure to pollens or pets. Exposure to non-allergic irritants such as cold air, chemicals, dust, and cigarette smoke will set off an asthma episode among yet another group of asthmatics. Even exercise can provoke bronchospasm in some asthmatics, particularly when airway inflammation is poorly controlled.

COPD, on the other hand, is a disease of lung destruction that has no cure. The lung tissue and small airways are destroyed by the COPD process, leading to chronic symptoms of breathlessness and cough. The typical on-and-off behaviour of asthma is not very prominent in COPD, except perhaps for the cycle of exertion and rest. For those with COPD, the symptoms are chronic and everyday for the rest of the patient's life.

At the present time, we don't have drug therapy that is specific for

FIGURE 15.2: COPD VERSUS ASTHMA

	COPD	ASTHMA
Age at onset	• usually diagnosed in early 50s or 60s	• may occur and be diagnosed at any age
History of allergy	• uncommon	• frequent
Smoking	• commonest cause	• not directly related, but may trigger attacks
Genetics	• probably important in determining susceptibility to lung damage from smoking • specifics not yet known	• important in determining risk for asthma • specifics not yet known
Clinical course of disease	• chronic, slowly progressive, regardless of therapy	• episodic symptoms • chronic illness may occur if asthma under-treated
Symptoms	• breathlessness, initially with exertion, progressing to chronic breathlessness • cough, phlegm	• attacks of breathlessness, chest tightness, wheeze, cough provoked by specific triggers
Response to bronchodilators	• unpredictable • anticholinergics often best (e.g., ipratropium)	• predictable • improvement with beta$_2$-agonists (e.g., salbutamol)
Response to inhaled corticosteroids	• rarely indicated	• virtually always indicated
Hypoxemia (an abnormally low concentration of oxygen in the blood)	• common in advanced disease	• uncommon except during severe attacks

COPD. Consequently, most of the drugs used for obstructive airway diseases are designed to treat asthma. Corticosteroids treat asthmatic eosinophilic inflammation. Beta$_2$-agonist bronchodilators treat asthmatic bronchospasm but can also help in COPD. A class of bronchodilators called anticholinergics can also help both asthma and COPD, but tend to be more effective for COPD. (There is more detailed information about drug therapy in chapter 10.)

Cystic Fibrosis

This inherited disease usually appears in infancy (although sometimes the diagnosis is not made until adulthood). It occurs more often in children of Caucasian ancestry than in other racial groups. In Canada, approximately three thousand adults and children have cystic fibrosis (CF). To be affected, a child must inherit a defective gene from both parents.

That defective gene makes it impossible for the body's cells to produce a certain protein. Without that protein, sodium and chloride collect in the cells, drying up the natural moisture in the lungs' airways. As a result, a dry, thick mucus accumulates in the lungs. In addition to causing a persistent cough, this mucus serves as a perfect trap for bacteria. And when bacteria collect in the lungs, infection is often the result. CF patients suffer from recurrent bouts of pneumonia and bronchitis. After many episodes of infection, the airways become permanently damaged and scarred, a condition known as bronchiectasis. Other body secretions are also affected, and many people with CF have trouble digesting food properly because of malfunction of the pancreas gland.

The lifespan for CF patients currently averages about thirty years. But ongoing developments in the treatment of this disease (many focusing on genetic engineering) and the advent of lung transplantation promise to add years to the lives of CF patients.

Bronchiectasis

As the name indicates, this disease affects the bronchi and bronchioles. Bronchiectasis is the permanent widening of these airways, and usually results from the damage caused by untreated or repeated bronchial infections, often dating from childhood.

A serious untreated infection can damage the airways, reducing their strength and resilience and leaving them permanently dilated. These widened airways become excellent hosts for bacteria-filled mucus that, in turn, produces more infections, setting up a vicious cycle. Because the lungs are damaged, the immune system can't fight off new infections of the bronchial tubes. These additional infections compound and continue the process, feeding the vicious cycle and further damaging

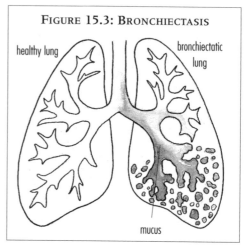

FIGURE 15.3: BRONCHIECTASIS

healthy lung

bronchiectatic lung

mucus

the lungs' airways. And on it goes unless the disease is diagnosed and treated.

Bronchiectasis usually causes chronic cough, shortness of breath, and fatigue. Because of the collection of mucus in the widened airways, the cough usually produces phlegm — a **productive cough**. The excessive coughing can irritate the fragile airways with the result that blood is spit up (called **hemoptysis**). Some people with bronchiectasis don't cough or produce phlegm regularly but have a "dry" type of bronchiectasis. For these people, the onset of cough, phlegm, or hemoptysis is usually a sign that the bronchial tubes have become infected, requiring treatment with antibiotics. Cystic fibrosis is one of the causes of bronchiectasis, but these days most bronchiectasis is seen in elderly people who suffered from tuberculosis or repeated pneumonias when they were young, many in the era before antibiotics were available. Hemoptysis can occasionally occur in COPD too, usually as a complication of a flare-up or pneumonia. But it may also be a sign that another smoking-related disease is present — lung cancer.

Lung Cancer

Just the words alone instill fear. We've all known someone who's died from the disease. Although lung cancer can occasionally be cured, this is not usually the case and, on average, the five-year survival rate is only about 50 percent.

Cancer is an abnormal growth of tissue — a tumour. A malignant

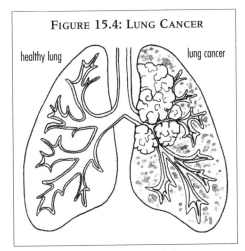

FIGURE 15.4: LUNG CANCER

healthy lung

lung cancer

tumour is one that spreads from its original site to other parts of the body. The tumour results from cells that begin to divide spontaneously, growing into an abnormal mass. These cancerous changes continue until the healthy cells in the tissue are outnumbered. The cancer takes hold and begins to spread.

We know that approximately 85 percent of lung cancer cases can be traced directly to cigarette smoking. But there are other causes of lung cancer, including exposure to second-hand smoke, asbestos, and other carcinogens.

Therapy for lung cancer is usually some combination of surgery, drugs (chemotherapy), or radiation therapy. Not all cancers are the same, and the type of cancerous cells will determine which treatment is best. For some types of lung cancer, surgical removal of the tumor is the best option, but only if the cancer is discovered early, before it has spread to other parts of the body and before it has become too large. This is a major operation and can be done only if the remaining lung tissue will be healthy enough to support life comfortably and if the person is healthy enough to tolerate the surgery. Sometimes surgery is combined with chemotherapy.

When drugs or surgery won't help, localized radiation therapy treatments may shrink the cancer and temporarily slow its growth, thus offering relief of symptoms. By far the best therapy for lung cancer is prevention, and that usually means quitting smoking or, better yet, never starting.

Bacterial and Viral Infections

Infections of the lungs and airways are a major cause of lung disease worldwide, and in some non-industrialized countries, chronic and recurrent infection of the lower respiratory tract can lead to permanent damage, including COPD and bronchiectasis. Lung infections occur in two basic forms: infections of the bronchial tubes, called **acute bronchitis,** and infection of the spongy portions of the lungs, called **pneumonia**. We've all had acute bronchitis at one time or another; usually we call it a chest cold. Pneumonia, on the other hand, is a bigger deal. It takes more out of you and can even be life threatening. Most lung infections are due to microorganisms called **viruses** or **bacteria**.

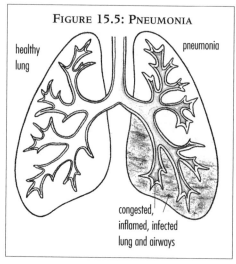

FIGURE 15.5: PNEUMONIA

healthy lung

pneumonia

congested, inflamed, infected lung and airways

Your mother called these microorganisms "germs." And her instructions to you (wash your hands, brush your teeth, don't pick your nose) are the standard hygienic recommendations still in force today to combat bacterial and viral infections. (You should always listen to your mother!)

If you were to stick your finger in your mouth and rub it over your gums and teeth, it would be covered with microscopic, single-celled bacteria. Your body is always filled with billions of bacteria. Similarly, the air, water, and soil around us are also filled with bacteria. Bacteria come in many different shapes and forms. The vast majority are completely harmless to humans. In fact, most are useful to us. We need bacteria in our intestines to break down our food as part of the digestion process, for example. But some bacteria, called **pathogens**, cause disease in humans.

Bacteria cause many diseases that affect the lungs: bacterial pneumonia, tuberculosis, and whooping cough, for example. In fact, you probably know some bacteria by name. *Streptococcus pneumoniae*, *Staphylococcus aureus*, and *Legionella* (Legionnaire's disease) are common bacteria that cause pneumonia.

For microorganisms to cause a lung infection, they must first enter your lungs. This can happen in countless way; breathing in droplets from someone else's sneeze, for example, is a common way to get a viral lung infection. The most common cause of bacterial pneumonia, however, is microaspiration of our *own* bacteria-laden oral secretions. We often breathe in minute amounts of our own oral secretions, especially when we sleep. (This is called microaspiration.) Once bacteria are in the body, they begin reproducing (in a few hours, a single bacterium can transform itself into a colony of 250,000). Usually, nothing bad happens because our defences against bacteria are healthy. Our immune system will seek out the bacteria we breathe in and kill them, preventing bacterial overgrowth and the development of pneumonia. But if our defences are weakened — by other diseases, malnutrition, cigarette smoking, or even by old age — the bacteria may not be killed off and pneumonia will take hold.

When fighting infection, the immune system kicks into high gear, increasing the blood flow to the infected area. This, in turn, causes inflammation (swelling, redness, and heat), which serves to flood the area with white blood cells that attempt to destroy the invading bacteria. But sometimes the body needs help. That's when **antibiotic drugs** can prove useful. Antibiotic drugs fight bacterial infection in different ways. Some simply kill the bacteria, others stop the bacteria from reproducing. They also vary in their targets. A **broad-spectrum antibiotic** fights a variety of bacteria. Other antibiotics are effective against only certain types of bacteria.

Antibiotics have no effect on viruses. This means that viral infections — a cold and influenza, for example — should not be treated with antibiotics. There's no point!

Like bacteria, not all viruses cause disease, but you've probably heard of some that do. HIV (human immunodeficiency virus) is the agent responsible for AIDS (acquired immune deficiency syndrome); herpes virus causes cold sores, chickenpox, and genital herpes; adenovirus is a common cause of colds; and influenza virus causes the flu. Viruses may also cause some cancers. Viruses can enter your body the same way that bacteria do. When a virus invades the cells of the body, your immune system goes into overdrive, bringing in white cells that work at devouring the virus. The body also produces **antibodies,** which destroy invading microorganisms.

In most cases, the immune system can beat down a viral infection within a few days. But the body can't respond in those people with weakened immune systems or where the virus is particularly virulent. In some cases, death is the result. In other cases, the weakened body becomes susceptible to a second wave of infection — this time often by bacteria. For people with COPD, this is a common sequence. A cold virus that seems to settle in the chest leads to a bacterial bronchitis or even pneumonia.

Antiviral drugs do exist but only for a few specific viruses, and they do not eliminate the viral infection, they only reduce it. Viruses are notoriously difficult to attack with drugs. Because they live inside the cells of the body, if you kill the virus, you damage the cell it's living in. Often the only way to deal with a viral infection is to treat the symptoms (drugs to reduce fever, for example) and wait for the immune system to kick in and rid your body of the virus naturally.

The best way of dealing with both viruses and bacteria is to protect yourself against the risk of infection. Don't get infected in the first place! In other words, practise prevention. Start by washing your hands and avoiding people who might have infectious diseases. Eat right, get adequate sleep, listen to the voice of your mother — use your common sense and look after your health. And get appropriate immunizations. For people with lung disease, vaccines against influenza and pneumonia are advisable. Talk with your doctor!

Restrictive Lung Diseases

Pulmonary Fibrosis

Perhaps you've heard of farmer's lung, asbestosis, sarcoidosis, or humidifier lung. These are all examples of pulmonary fibrosis, or **interstitial lung disease**. "Fibrosis" means a thickening and scarring of tissue. "Interstitial" refers to the supporting tissues of the lung in the interstitium region located between the airways and the alveoli. In some countries, pulmonary fibrosis is referred to as **fibrosing alveolitis,** or inflammation of the alveoli leading to fibrosis.

Fibrosis in the lung means that alveoli are destroyed and replaced by scar tissue. The small capillaries of the interstitium that keep blood circulating around the alveoli are also destroyed by scar tissue. Because of this destruction, the patient loses

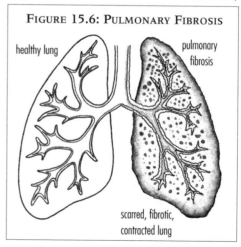

FIGURE 15.6: PULMONARY FIBROSIS

healthy lung

pulmonary fibrosis

scarred, fibrotic, contracted lung

the use of large parts of the lung, resulting in shortness of breath, a deficiency of oxygen in the blood and, in advanced cases, secondary failure of the right chambers of the heart due to pulmonary hypertension (similar to what happens in advanced COPD).

But what causes this scarring? The common names for this spectrum of disorders speak volumes. The causes of pulmonary fibrosis can often be identified: mouldy hay and barn dust for farmer's lung; exposure to asbestos for asbestosis; humidifiers contaminated with mould for humidifier lung. However, about half the time we don't know the cause of the fibrosis. In these cases, the terms **idiopathic fibrosis** or **cryptogenic fibrosing alveolitis** are used to describe our ignorance.

Here's what happens. Foreign substances — anything from bird droppings to particles of sand to mould in a hot tub to cocaine snorted up the nose — are inhaled into the lungs. These substances injure the airways and the alveoli. The immune system goes into overdrive, attempting to repair the initial injury. But instead of making things better, somehow the repair process causes widespread inflammation of the lungs that eventually leads to extensive scarring or fibrosis, permanently damaging the airways, alveoli, and capillaries. And just like that mark on your knee from a childhood injury, a scar is for life.

Often the first sign of pulmonary fibrosis is shortness of breath or a persistent dry cough. It's an easy symptom to ignore initially. Patients usually respond by adopting a more sedentary lifestyle and chalking up breathlessness to aging. Breathlessness is often accompanied by a tight, dry, persistent cough that doesn't produce much phlegm. Treatment for fibrosis is not very successful. Corticosteroids and other immunosuppressive drugs occasionally help, but for the most part treatment is supportive (oxygen therapy and rehabilitation, for example). Because of this, lung transplantation is a treatment that is available for pulmonary fibrosis, but only in certain select cases.

Pleural Diseases

If you imagine the lungs as a set of sponges inside a glass jar, the sponge is the lung, the glass jar is the chest cavity. The lung sponge and the inside surface of the chest wall are both covered with a thin lining called the **pleura**, which is like the peel of an orange, only much thinner. In between the sponge and the jar is a thin space called the **pleural space**. The pleura are very pain-sensitive, and when inflamed cause chest pain, or **pleurisy**, a sharp pain that is made worse by deep breathing or coughing.

Pleurisy can complicate an infection of the lungs — pneumonia, for example. The inflamed pleura can weep fluid into the pleural space, causing what is known as a **pleural effusion** (like water in the glass jar). When an effusion is large, it can interfere with breathing and must be drained by a tube. The pleura can also thicken when they are affected by a particular cancer called **mesothelioma**, which is usually caused by heavy exposure to asbestos.

Diseases of the pleura restrict lung function and impede breathing either by causing pain or by thickening the lining of the lung, making breathing hard work, and causing even more breathlessness.

Chest Wall Problems

The most common chest wall restriction is caused by a big gut. This is one of the reasons people with COPD are encouraged to achieve an ideal weight, if possible. Losing the big gut reduces the work of breathing that is already in overdrive because of COPD. Arthritis, which has the effect of stiffening the ribs, is another cause of chest wall restriction.

As you can see, the lungs can be affected by many different types of diseases. But by far the two most common conditions leading to chronic lung disease are the obstructive diseases — asthma and COPD. Currently we have reasonably good therapy for asthma. For COPD, however, apart from controlling symptoms, we really don't have that much to offer.

To see what the future might hold for new COPD treatments, move on to chapter 16.

16

A Brave New World —
Hope for the Future

"Yes, I'm afraid," begins Lorraine. "Fear is always part of my life. Every day I wake up, I'm grateful to be here another day to think of my future. So, if I get a second chance, I'm going for it." Lorraine is struggling with advanced emphysema. Her condition might realistically be described as "end stage." She must take continuous oxygen therapy and becomes breathless with even the simplest activities. Even a minor cold can be life-threatening for her. An amazing woman, she works diligently at keeping herself active, productive, and upbeat. One reason Lorraine copes so well is the support of her husband, Larry, who has moved heaven and earth to make things easier for her. Another reason is her hope for the future.

Lorraine has been on the lung transplant list at the London Health Sciences Centre in London, Ontario, for more than a year. She's endured a couple of serious flare-ups recently and is waiting for the call telling her that a new lung is waiting — that her second chance has arrived. A new lung is what it will take for Lorraine because today we do not have the ability to reverse the COPD process and restore lung function to normal. We can't cure COPD.

The best hope we currently have to change the relentless downhill progression of advanced COPD is to try to stop its major cause — cigarette smoking. As we discussed in chapter 9, we know that quitting smoking often slows the rate of lung function decline that occurs with aging in susceptible smokers. This makes sense, since the chemicals from cigarette smoke will no longer be present to stimulate the protease enzymes and the neutrophils responsible for the lung destruction and mucus hypersecretion of COPD.

None of the drugs currently available to treat COPD can slow its progression — they can only treat the symptoms. What we really need are some "smart" drugs that can slow, prevent, or even reverse the lung damage that comes with COPD. To develop smart therapy, we need to get smarter ourselves by fostering a better understanding of all the molecular and chemical reactions that occur in the airways of people who go on to develop COPD.

The good news is that a lot of sophisticated research is being done to answer these crucial questions. Progress is definitely being made. Although many years of research and development lie ahead, it certainly looks as if we (or at least our children and grandchildren) can look forward to new treatments that will be able to slow or even halt altogether the destructive process of COPD. It's important to continue these efforts, since the triggers for developing COPD — smoking, air pollution, and chronic infection of the airways, for example — will never entirely disappear.

There is some hope for the present, too. Bronchodilator medications can reduce some of the breathlessness of COPD, especially if adequate doses are taken. Ipratropium, for example, should probably be taken in relatively large doses — twelve to sixteen puffs per day — to get the maximum benefit. Although such a high dosage is safe, it is tedious. The once-a-day anticholinergic bronchodilator tiotropium (Spiriva) promises to be helpful in this regard. Newer developments in theophyllines and drugs that act on dopamine receptors in the airways are also in the works.

One of the most effective anti-breathlessness therapies available for COPD, however, doesn't involve drugs at all. The physical conditioning, coping skills, and confidence building that can result from a pulmonary rehabilitation program can be one of the most effective ways to bring disabling breathlessness under control. Not everyone with COPD has access to a rehabilitation program, and for others, coexisting health problems may limit the benefits they could achieve from rehabilitation. Yet even after taking all the drugs and doing all the exercises, many people with advanced COPD remain severely breathless and disabled. Is there *anything* that can be done to help these folks?

This is where surgical therapy for COPD has been advocated. Usually we think of surgery as a therapy used to fix something that has gone bad in our bodies and that must be removed — like replacing worn tires on your car. In many ways, surgical therapy for COPD is exactly like that; only in this case, the worn-out components are your lungs.

It's difficult to imagine surgically repairing the multitudinous holes caused throughout the lung tissue by emphysema. It simply couldn't be done. But there are some circumstances where surgery may help ease the burden of breathlessness in the advanced emphysematous forms of COPD. One of these is the surgical removal of large, localized, over-distended pouches of lung tissue called **bullae** (pronounced "bull-eye"). A bulla is like a thin weak spot in a balloon that bulges out excessively as the balloon is inflated — like a local patch of severe emphysema. Occasionally, bullae can become so large that they take up too much space within the chest cavity and compress the rest of the lungs. The result is an extreme degree of hyperinflation, which hinders normal breathing and results in constant, disabling breathlessness. By surgically removing the bullae, the local hyperinflation can be reduced and the pressure taken off the surrounding lungs, restoring more normal function and reducing breathlessness. The bullae situation doesn't arise too often in COPD, but it's worth recognizing, since this is one condition where surgery can provide dramatic benefits.

If you understand the principles behind surgery for bullae in COPD, you'll have no trouble understanding the rationale for the latest attempt to treat COPD surgically — **lung volume reduction surgery (LVRS)**. You may have read in the newspapers about this so-called surgical cure for emphysema.

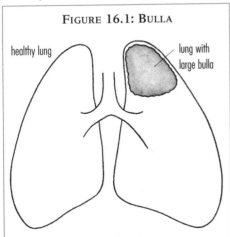

FIGURE 16.1: BULLA

healthy lung

lung with large bulla

The media hype is unfortunate, since the vast majority of people with COPD encouraged by the news of LVRS will not benefit from this dramatic operation.

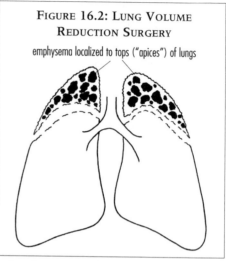

FIGURE 16.2: LUNG VOLUME REDUCTION SURGERY

emphysema localized to tops ("apices") of lungs

For most people with the predominantly emphysematous form of COPD, the "lung holes" occur diffusely throughout both lungs — like Swiss cheese (see Figure 4.5). There's nothing that can be done surgically to fix this, except total replacement of the lungs — lung transplantation. Occasionally, however, in some people with emphysema, the lung holes tend to be clustered mainly at the periphery of the lungs and especially at the tops, or apices, of the lungs. If this is the case, the many emphysematous holes effectively act like a large bulla, causing excessive hyperinflation and displacement of less damaged lung tissue, contributing to disabling breathlessness. The surgical solution to this problem is obvious — cut out the bad bits. Just like pruning the dead portions on the edges of a hedge, lung volume reduction surgery cuts away the clusters of emphysematous holes at the tops of the lungs. The surgery reduces breathlessness by reducing hyperinflation and allowing the remainder of the lungs to re-expand more normally.

Although this new surgery is very promising, it is certainly not a true cure for emphysema — the underlying emphysematous process remains unaltered. And although LVRS will help only a minority of people with COPD, the results can be dramatic when it does work, reducing breathlessness, increasing exercise capacity, and thus improving quality of life and sometimes life expectancy.

LVRS is a fairly new procedure, so data on how it affects mortality in COPD are somewhat scarce. In one trial, however, the LVRS increased the chance of being alive three years after qualifying for the surgery from 64 percent for those who did not get the surgery to 82 percent for those who did. If you have emphysema and wonder whether LVRS would be helpful for you, your doctor will first need to order a CT scan of your lungs to see whether there is enough localized emphysema to make the surgery practical.

The other dramatic form of surgery that can help people with advanced COPD is lung transplantation. We have the ability to transplant one lung, two lungs, or even two lungs and the heart for people with far-advanced COPD. This is drastic and dramatic stuff. Even when only one lung is replaced, the improvements in symptoms and sense of well-being can be remarkable. With single-lung transplants, one diseased lung is left in place, but the new good lung can more than compensate. The COPD in the remaining bad lung does not spread to the new lung. It is understood, of course, that the recipient will remain a non-smoker.

Estimating any survival benefit for lung transplantation in COPD is difficult. Recipients of lung transplants face an ongoing risk that the transplanted lung will be rejected, and eventually some form of rejection does occur in most people. For this and other reasons, to date there has been no clear-cut survival benefit shown for lung transplantation in COPD. However, lung transplantation appears to significantly reduce breathlessness, and improve endurance and overall quality of life, which justifies it as a valuable rescue therapy for end-stage COPD in certain people.

People who qualify for lung transplantation must be relatively young (usually under sixty-five) and must remain as fit as possible — some transplantation programs require enrolment in an ongoing pulmonary rehabilitation program. The decision to transplant is not arrived at lightly. Very few lungs become available for transplantation.

Perhaps in the future — when cloning technology improves so animals (likely pigs) can be bred as donors — lung availability will improve considerably. Today, however, lungs for transplantation are scarce. Only the best potential recipients are chosen, and the selection process can be arduous, both physically and emotionally. Even once you are accepted and have a coveted spot on the waiting list, the strain can be considerable. Will I get a lung? When? Will I live long enough to get a lung? Will I stay healthy enough to still qualify? On top of these and other issues is the emotional and philosophical dilemma of waiting for someone to die so that you might live longer. Each person will handle this emotional situation differently.

Lorraine and her husband, Larry, are well acquainted with the emotional roller coaster of the lung transplantation waiting list. "In the past year, I've been at my wit's end several times," says Lorraine. The couple, together with their two grown children, spent a lot of time discussing whether Lorraine should ask to be placed on the list. In the end, the decision proved to be easy for all of them. "The alternative is worse," explains Larry. Their decision was reinforced when Lorraine and Larry met Claudette, a woman who'd recently undergone a lung transplant that gave her back a significant degree of good health.

Both Lorraine and Larry talk about the day-to-day strain of waiting — waiting for the pager Larry wears on his belt to sound with the news that a new lung is waiting for Lorraine in London. "We work hard at thinking about other things but we can never forget about it," says Lorraine. Both are resigned to the possibility that the new lung may never arrive for Lorraine: "I feel that if my number doesn't come up, it doesn't come up." These lessons have been hard learned.

Lorraine has endured serious disappointments during her time on the waiting list. A misdiagnosis of lung cancer pushed her off the list for a few weeks. "I was very angry and depressed, but we worked hard to keep on an even keel." Larry has the task of keeping in constant contact with the transplant coordinator in London, informing him of any changes in Lorraine's condition — good and bad — that might affect her chances in the "lung lottery."

Surgical therapy for advanced COPD is hopeful, but very few people with COPD will qualify for any of the surgical treatments we have discussed. Is there any hope for those who don't qualify? At this time, there are really only two options. One is to find some way of accepting the situation and making the best of it by concentrating on preserving the best quality of life possible for as long as possible. In the final analysis, this approach is a fact of life for all of us, whether we have a chronic illness like COPD or not. Each of us will manage this in our own way.

For those with advanced COPD who cannot or will not sit back and "wait for the end," the only other option is to consider mechanical ventilation in the home. As COPD advances, the disease imposes a tremendous increase in the work of breathing and, thus, on the muscles of breathing. Eventually, the breathing muscles can't keep up the work required. They fatigue and fail. When this occurs, lung ventilation falls off and the carbon dioxide level in the blood increases to dangerous levels — ultimately death ensues. (This same sort of thing can occur during COPD flare-ups, when the patient requires a temporary period of mechanical ventilation.) Long-term mechanical ventilation at home to rest the breathing muscles for people with stable end-stage COPD is possible. The machine is often used at night to, in effect, "recharge the batteries" by resting the breathing muscles. More comfortable, unassisted breathing is then possible during the daytime. Home ventilation can be administered either through a non-invasive tight-fitting mask or by a short tracheostomy tube inserted surgically through the neck.

Only a few people with COPD, however, are suitable candidates for home ventilation. It can be a very labour-intensive and costly enterprise, requiring significant amounts of support. For those who do qualify and take the task on, only about half stick with it for any reasonable length of time. Nevertheless, this "last-ditch" treatment can ease symptoms and perhaps add both some meaningful quality of life and precious time for some people.

The last words belong to a brave woman who has faced down death and come out the victor. Lorraine says her days are long. She's working hard, staying in physical shape, walking on her treadmill, shopping with Larry, keeping her mind and body busy. But she's waiting and wondering. "What if I could play golf again? What if I could be independent again? What if? In the meantime, I keep going. I've got to do what I've got to do."

Afterword

Courage does not always march to airs blown by a bugle; is not always wrought out of the fabric ostentation wears.

FRANCES RODMAN

*D*uring the writing of this book, we got to know some wonderful people — smart, funny, kind men and women. Most are married, a couple divorced. Most have kids. They worked as nurses, teachers, secretaries, engineers, accountants. Ordinary folks. But disease — a challenging chronic disease — sent the lives of our group of eleven off the ordinary path and into a difficult new reality. In facing the challenge of living with COPD, all eleven have shown their courage. To a person, they wear their courage privately and, if you met them in the street, you'd probably think them quite ordinary. They're not.

In the time between the writing of *Every Breath I Take* and its publication, two of our group of eleven died. Janet died of emphysema on March 26, 2000. Edgar died of pneumonia on April 5, 2000.

Lorraine continues to wait for the call telling her that a new lung is ready for her.

Rick Hodder
November 16, 2000

What Your Doctors Are Reading about COPD

You've learned a lot about COPD by reading this book. We know that some of you — like Raymond — want to know even more. In chapter 5 we listed some resources you can use to further expand your knowledge of COPD. Here we list some recently published guidelines for physicians that help them do their best for patients with COPD. If you're interested in this level of detail, your library can help you access these articles from the medical literature.

American Thoracic Society official statement. "Standards for the diagnosis and care of patients with chronic obstructive pulmonary disease." *American Journal of Respiratory and Critical Care Medicine* 1995; 152: S77–S120.

British Thoracic Society. "Guidelines for the management of chronic obstructive pulmonary disease." *Thorax* 1997; 52 (suppl. 5): S1–S28.

European Respiratory Society consensus statement. "Optimal assessment and management of chronic obstructive pulmonary disease (COPD)." *European Respiratory Journal* 1995; 8: 1398–420.

Canadian Respiratory Review Panel. *Guidelines for the Treatment of Chronic Obstructive Pulmonary Disease (COPD)*. Toronto: Medication Use Management Guidelines Clearing House, 1998.

Canadian Thoracic Society Workshop Group. Guidelines for the assessment and management of chronic obstructive pulmonary disease. *Canadian Medical Association Journal* 1992; 147 (4): 420–28.

Index